T0231404

MCQs in Geriatric Medicine for Postgraduate Examinations

ROGER GABRIEL

*Emeritus Consultant Physician in General and Renal Medicine,
St Mary's Hospital, Paddington, London and
Northwick Park Hospital, Harrow, Middlesex
Locum Consultant Physician, Department of Medicine for
the Elderly, Addenbrooke's Hospital, Cambridge*

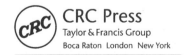

CRC Press
Taylor & Francis Group
Boca Raton London New York

CRC Press is an imprint of the
Taylor & Francis Group, an **informa** business

Radcliffe Publishing Ltd
33–41 Dallington Street
London
EC1V 0BB
United Kingdom

www.radcliffepublishing.com

British Library Cataloguing in Publication Data

A catalogue record for this book is available from the British Library.

ISBN-13: 978 184619 576 1

The paper used for the text pages of this book
is FSC® certified. FSC (The Forest Stewardship
Council®) is an international network to promote
responsible management of the world's forests.

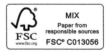

Typeset by Darkriver Design, Auckland, New Zealand

Contents

Preface

The idea for this book occurred whilst I was writing the Diploma of Geriatric Medicine (DGM) examination in February 2011. The range and level of the questions then had become apparent – very few are published – but of these few, some were recycled in the paper. After the examination I scribbled down the 30-odd questions I recalled – they are scattered across the following pages – began writing these MCQs and happily found Radcliffe Publishing to be most accommodating.

Geriatric medicine has expanded from general internal medicine having developed a range of additional facts, approaches, social, ethical, managerial and team efforts. These topics are emphasised in the following MCQs. The overall proportions of topics are roughly those as suggested by the Royal College of Physicians, London but I have added more questions proportional to the importance of some topics. The vignettes are, in the main, based on actual patients I have managed over the past four years. Drug therapy in the elderly is frequently mismanaged and provides instructive MCQ material.

This book is for postgraduate doctors who need to succeed in elderly medicine-biased MCQs – candidates for the DGM and similar diplomas, registrars in geriatric medicine reading for their Specialty Certificates and for Part I MRCP candidates because of their need to have a decent grasp of this rapidly increasing branch of medicine in terms of information, number of patients and cost to the State.

Two disclaimers – drug doses are mentioned in places and I believe them to be correct but this book does not have *BNF*-like authority. Second, I think the text is factually correct but errors cannot be excluded. If anyone has the energy to point them out I will correct them in the next printing.

It has been fun putting together these questions and answers. I hope you will enjoy them. When you have cracked all 350, you will have the MCQ examiners on toast.

Roger Gabriel
Cambridge
March 2012

About the author

Roger Gabriel qualified, trained and practiced in London. Last century he took early retirement from the NHS and after working in Zimbabwe and two spells for the Ministry of Defence he became a persistent, peripatetic locum in general, geriatric and acute medicine. He plans to continue as such until his permanent retirement in 2016.

For wonderful Wendy, my wife

Classification of cases

The various sub-divisions of the discipline are scattered across the text but for those who wish to pursue specific themes, here is a classification by topic. The numbers refer to questions, not pages.

Cardiovascular
58, 67, 80, 113, 116, 124, 129, 158, 175, 201, 211, 214, 225, 238, 242, 248, 261, 275, 291, 301, 314, 316, 322, 329, 332, 349

Drugs and therapeutics
6, 30, 42, 57, 64, 66, 77, 94, 106, 120, 126, 138, 140, 154, 163, 170, 174, 184, 198, 217, 234, 245, 253, 260, 269, 313, 319, 328, 341

Gastroenterology
5, 14, 26, 33, 62, 70, 123, 125, 161, 191, 208, 226, 235, 249, 257, 262, 312, 325, 335

Haematology and oncology
1, 10, 21, 24, 39, 60, 78, 102, 149, 204, 318, 350

Infectious disease
72, 108, 139, 147, 153, 172, 180, 202, 205, 215, 222, 252, 296, 302, 304, 334, 343

Legal topics
45, 55, 75, 88, 117, 168, 183, 192, 196, 207, 213, 231, 237, 251, 287, 320

Mental dysfunction
44, 51, 59, 68, 73, 81, 99, 103, 111, 137, 176, 179, 189, 259, 264, 265, 284, 297, 317, 342, 346

Metabolic
8, 17, 35, 40, 93, 96, 101, 127, 141, 152, 169, 177, 182, 186, 206, 229, 239, 254, 285, 298, 305, 306, 308, 315, 333, 337

Miscellaneous

9, 13, 16, 22, 38, 43, 47, 54, 71, 82, 91, 92, 100, 105, 107, 110, 115, 130, 143, 146, 151, 155, 162, 167, 193, 209, 216, 243, 250, 279, 295

Mouth, ears and eyes

12, 20, 31, 32, 34, 65, 84, 114, 144, 145, 164, 166, 188, 194, 212, 218, 240, 256, 280, 289, 293, 340

Musculo-skeletal

4, 19, 27, 29, 37, 41, 74, 98, 112, 118, 122, 134, 135, 160, 190, 221, 224, 236, 267, 281, 311, 327

Neurology

2, 18, 23, 25, 76, 79, 86, 90, 109, 119, 132, 157, 171, 199, 210, 227, 232, 258, 268, 270, 276, 278, 288, 290, 292, 299, 309, 310, 321, 324, 331, 347

Renal tract

3, 28, 36, 63, 104, 121, 133, 159, 173, 178, 187, 241, 255, 272, 282, 294, 330, 339

Respiratory

50, 52, 69, 83, 89, 131, 150, 165, 197, 219, 244, 247, 266, 277, 300, 323

Skin and nails

7, 11, 46, 48, 49, 87, 95, 156, 195, 200, 230, 233, 286, 303, 336, 345

Social topics

15, 53, 56, 61, 97, 128, 136, 142, 181, 185, 203, 223, 228, 230, 246, 263, 271, 273, 274, 283, 307, 326, 338, 344, 348

Reference range of laboratory variables

This list of laboratory variables is far from comprehensive, including only those concentrations that are used in the MCQs. I have tended to smooth out values for ease of use and have not quoted separate ranges for men and women.

Chemical pathology

sodium	135–145 mmol/L
potassium	3.5–5.0 mmol/L
urea	2.5–7.5 mmol/L
creatinine	60–100 µmol/L
eGFR	5– 90 ml/min
calcium	2.0–2.5 mmol/L
phosphate	0.8–1.5 mmol/L
urate	200–420 µmol/L
cholesterol	< 4.5 mmol/L
cortisol morning, fasting	135–700 nmol/L
creatine phosphokinase, CK	< 350 U/L
C-reactive protein, CRP	< 10 mg/L
digoxin	1.0–2.0 µg/L
free thyroxine, FT4	70–140 mmol/L
glucose fasting (normal)	4.2–5.6 mmol/L
fasting (diabetic)	> 7.0 mmol/L
HbA_{1c}	< 6.5% (45 mmol/mol)
albumin	35–55 g/L
alanine aminotransferase, ALT	10–50 U/L
aspartate aminotransferase, AST	10–50 U/L
alkaline phosphatase, AP	40–125 U/L
gamma-glutamyl transferase, γGT	10–50 U/L
bilirubin	2–17 umol/L
thyroid stimulating hormone, TSH	0.15–3.5 mU/L
prostatate specific antigen, PSA	0.0–6.0 µg/L
B naturetic peptide, BNP	< 400 ng/L

Haematology

Hb	12–18 g/dl
red blood cell count	$3.5–5.5 \times 10^{12}$/L
MCV	80–100 fl
MCHC	27–32 pg
reticulocyte count	0.8–2.0% of red cells
wbc	$3.5–10.0 \times 10^9$/L
neutrophils	40–70%
platelets	$150–400 \times 10^9$/L
international normalised ratio, INR	< 1.1
activated partial thromboplastin time, APPT	25–35 sec
B_{12}	20–750 pmol/L
ferritin	30–250 µg/L

Urine

random sample sodium	10–80 mmol/L
albumin/creatinine ratio (acr)	< 3 mg/mmol
protein/creatinine ratio (pcr)	< 45 mg/mmol
osmolality	200–800 mOsm/kg water

Questions 1–350

1   An asymptomatic man of 75 years had some routine blood tests upon joining a new surgery. Results:

Hb	11.2
MCV	114
reticulocyte count	0.3%
platelets	89
wbc	2.9
creatinine	85

What was the likely diagnosis?
A   vitamin B_{12} deficiency
B   haemolysis
C   aplastic anaemia
D   iron deficiency
E   myelofibrosis

2   Which one of the following is an infrequent feature of a transient ischaemic attack (TIA)?
A   loss of consciousness
B   aphasia or dysphasia
C   amaurosis fugax
D   hemiparesis
E   hemisensory disturbance

3   An elderly person consulted her doctor because for many months she was 'always wet'. From which of the following list of drug groups could a suitable prescription be chosen?
A   an α-blocker
B   an anticholinergenic
C   an antimuscarinic
D   a 5α-reductase inhibitor
E   none of these

4   What is the most likely low energy impact pelvic bone damage in an elderly person?
A a superior ramus
B an inferior ramus
C both
D separation of the pubic symphysis
E a sacral insufficiency fracture

5   George Gross, bed bound but only 7 years away from the Queen's telegram, was admitted to a community hospital to allow his wife a period of respite. Over a week he developed a distended, tympanic abdomen. There was anorexia and some retching.

What was the likely explanation?
A ascites
B aerophagia
C constipation
D small bowel obstruction
E large bowel volvulus

6   Emily Green attended her doctor on account of her husband of 60 years, who had been disturbing her sleep because of his involuntary twitching and moving of his legs for the first hours after they retired to bed. The patient's eyes were sunken and papillary responses to light and accommodation were slow. Deep tendon reflexes were absent in both legs. Edward Green's results:

Hb	10.2
MCV	88
ferritin	100
CRP	7
CK	128

Which was the drug of choice to help the Greens?
A ferrous sulphate
B quinine
C levodopa
D zopiclone
E ropinirole

7 Tom 'Banting' Best celebrated 60 years of insulin therapy on his 78th birthday. He had developed a deep ulcer on the base of his 5th right metatarsal.

Examination: ulcer 1.5 cm deep, punched out with regular edges; skin: pale, cool and hairless; nails: atrophic; no pulses palpable below femorals; capillary refill time 5 seconds.

What treatment should not be used?
A skin grafting
B tight diabetic control
C compression bandaging
D expert podiatry
E prescription of vitamin C and zinc supplements

8 A woman of 80 years with diabetes had periods of confusion. She was registered blind due to retinopathy. A district nurse visited each day at 7.30 a.m. to measure blood glucose and give 20 units of insulin glargine. BM figures ranged from 7.7 to 10 mmol/L; HbA_{1c} 6.55% (48 mmol/mol).

What was needed to be done?
A increase glargine by 4 units
B decrease glargine by 2 units
C organise a dementia screen
D obtain a more extensive blood sugar profile
E withhold glargine and assess in 2 days

9 Which of the following is one of the 'Four Giants of Geriatric Medicine'?
A constipation
B recurrent urinary infection
C repeated falls
D pressure ulcers
E iatrogenic illness

10 A note was posted to Mrs White's GP requesting 'a course of iron tablets' on account of a 'hypochromic microcytic blood film' which had been found by chance. Ferrous fumarate 322 mg twice daily was prescribed. Three months later the results from a blood film were unchanged.

What was the least likely explanation?
A coeliac disease
B pharyngeal pouch
C thalassaemia trait
D lack of compliance
E angiodysplasia

11 A 91-year-old woman had itching around her 'front bottom'. Which of the following was an unlikely cause?

A atrophic vulvitis

B vulval dystrophy

C vulval carcinoma

D pubic lice

E 2nd degree uterine prolapse

12 Ten years on from retirement the widowed Harry Hearhard became depressed and withdrawn because the once enjoyable, friendly, familiar, noisy environment at the 'Legion' and his bingo club made clear hearing increasingly difficult. Some sounds were too soft, others uncomfortably loud. High-pitched sounds became inaudible. He had to adjust the volume of his radio and TV carefully so that they were not uncomfortable to hear.

What had happened?

A bi-lateral impacted dry wax in both external auditory canals

B Ménière's disease

C dry chronic otitis media

D otosclerosis

E presbycusis

13 Regarding informal carers, which of the following is wrong?

A the care receiver may be entitled to claim an Attendance Allowance (AA)

B the higher rate AA is means tested

C carers may risk their health while caring for a family member

D carers' average age is 60 to 70+ years

E some carers are teenagers

14 Flo Smith, born 1930, was well. Every day she took a compound preparation of aspirin and dipyridamole. Which of the following was not an indication to refer her for colonic endoscopy?

A a great-niece of 38 had recently died from a disseminated sigmoid carcinoma

B a one-year history of irritable bowel syndrome

C pneumaturia

D a chance finding of a MCV of 75

E 4 months of variable diarrhoea

15 Which one of the following is incorrect?
  A the UK population is about 61 million
  B the average woman of 65 years can expect to live to 85
  C in ten years' time a 65-year-old woman will have a life expectancy of 23 years
  D since 1980 the population > 65 years old has increased by circa 30%
  E between 2000 and 2010 the largest actual population growth was in the fourth quintile of life

16 For a month an 83-year-old-woman was 'off colour', had severe morning headaches, a tender scalp and painful mastication. Repeated attacks of amaurosis fugax propelled her to her general practitioner. She had had typical migraine which ceased at the time of her menopause. At 69 she had experienced a neck whiplash in a horse riding accident.

What was the most likely cause of her headache?
  A a brain tumour
  B cranial arteritis
  C recurrence of migraine
  D herpes zoster of the 2nd division of the Vth cranial nerve
  E cervical spondylitis

17 An 85-year-old woman was taken to her GP by her daughter because of 'palpitations'. She was tired, had some weight loss but was generally well.

Examination: pulse irregular at circa 100 bpm; BP 134/90; not in heart failure; fine tremor.

What single investigation was appropriate?
  A an ECG
  B exercise tolerance test
  C full blood count
  D thyroid function
  E B natriuretic peptide assay

18 When should treatment of a 71-year-old man with freshly diagnosed typical idiopathic Parkinson's disease (PD) begin treatment?
  A after he has had a chat with a fellow PD patient
  B when the informed person is 'ready' to start
  C as soon as the diagnosis is made
  D to improve micrographia
  E when instability becomes an increasing hazard

19 Which of the following is a feature of fibromyalgia?
  A characterised by proximal muscle pain
  B has an equal male:female incidence
  C characterised by multiple tender points
  D affects about 10% of people over 70 years
  E may evolve to a large joint arthritis

20 Which is the commonest cause of adult blind registration in the UK?
  A type I diabetes
  B glaucoma
  C retinitis pigmentosa
  D malignant hypertension
  E age-related macular degeneration

21 Korean war veteran Brigadier Sir Julian Blimp GC (retired), ex-Eton, Sandhurst and the Guards, consulted his Harley Street physician because of periods of dizziness and fainting – 'can't keep me parade legs, dontcher know?' Alcohol intake: 50 to 55 units weekly. He took no medicines.

Examination: BP 142/59; 108/48; 138/54 – lying; standing; and standing for 3 minutes, respectively.

Haematology: MCV 76

What was a likely diagnosis?
  A liver disease
  B gastritis
  C myelofibrosis
  D megaloblastosis
  E duodenal ulcer

22 85-year-old 'Crasher' Tumble attended a Falls Clinic because he had had fallen repeatedly over the previous six weeks. He used a delta rollator.

What was untrue of Mr Tumble and similar people?
  A falls are more frequent in men
  B adequate help requires a multidisciplinary team
  C multiple falls often lead to institutionalisation
  D falls usually have several causes
  E the wearing of bifocal spectacles is a risk factor

23 At Easter 2008 Dr Jill Fenton, once a spry 80-year-old retired Oxbridge Classics don, found that the *Times* crossword took over 15 minutes (previously 7–10 minutes) to complete and by mid-2012 she could solve no more than three clues. Over the same time span she became incontinent of urine.

Examination: unsteady with a broad-based gait.

What was the likely diagnosis?
A Lewy Body disease
B Wilson's disease
C Parkinsonism
D Alzheimer's dementia
E normal pressure hydrocephalus

24 Dai Llewellyn, an ex-coal miner, was 'not myself since my wife died' – some 18 months previously. 'I am feeling my age' – 80 years. He had persistent left upper quadrant discomfort.

Examination: an easily palpable, firm spleen.

Blood test results:

Hb	9.3
MCV	105
platelets	55
wbc	2.6
blood film:	leukoerythroblastic picture with tear drop poikilocytes
bone marrow:	dry tap

What was the most likely diagnosis?
A iron deficiency
B myelofibrosis
C early aplastic anaemia
D aleukaemic leukaemia
E lymphoma

25 Applying the Framingham Heart Study data to 77-year-old men who have had an ischaemic stroke, which is the most common outcome at six months?
A some degree of hemiparesis
B needing assistance to walk
C unable to live independently
D aphasic
E needing enteral feeding

26 A widowed 79-year-old man whose behaviour had led his children to disown him was brought by the police to an A & E department. He had been sleeping in a park, was unkempt and uncommunicative.

Examination: bruised and scratched; icteric; tender right thorax; BP 179/108.

Investigations: chest x-ray: three fractured ribs.

Hb	9.9
MCV	107
ferritin	505
wbc	15.9
CRP	21
bilirubin	48
alk phos	156
ALT	250

What was the diagnosis?
A obstructive jaundice
B Diogenes syndrome
C alcoholic liver disease
D hepatocellular carcinoma
E last onset haemochromatosis

27 Which is the most commonly affected section of the spine to be involved by metastatic cord compression?
A cervical
B thoracic
C lumbar
D sacral
E diffuse

28 Apart from obstructive uropathy, which is the most common cause of end-stage renal failure in an elderly UK population?
A hypertension
B reflux nephropathy
C diabetes
D glomerulonephritis
E polycystic renal disease

29 Which one statement concerning gout is incorrect?
   A urate crystals in an acute joint are both extracellular and intracellular
   B the first stage of the metabolic condition is an asymptomatic hyperuricaemia
   C under polarised light the needle-shaped urate crystals are negatively birefringent
   D initially gout is a self-limiting monoarticular joint condition
   E most elderly patients need allopurinol 300 mg daily

30 After 10 days of treatment with imipramine 75 mg daily, 82-year-old Mr Williams returned to his GP to report new onset of sweating and rapid heart rate. Established long-term medications: aspirin, omeprazole, beta-histine, perindopril and simvastatin.

blood results:		
	wbc	10.2
	Na$^+$	138
	K$^+$	4.3
	Ca^{2+}	2.47
	TSH	0.45
	CRP	3

   What was the cause of the symptoms?
   A urinary tract infection
   B drug related
   C tuberculosis
   D lymphoma
   E anxiety

31 Concerning tinnitus, which of the following is not correct?
   A may be caused by aspirin
   B may accompany deafness
   C is not a causal feature of presbycusis
   D may comprise musical or other meaningful sounds
   E may be caused by parenteral furosemide

32 What is the commonest tumour of the eyelid in elderly people?
   A sebaceous cell carcinoma
   B basal cell carcinoma
   C actinic keratosis
   D squamous cell carcinoma
   E metastatic carcinoma

33 Twelve weeks after a 10-day course of eradication therapy (omeprazole + clarithromycin + metronidazole) for *Helicobacter pylori*, Ethel Brown no longer had duodenal ulcer symptoms but remained IgG positive for *H pylori*.

What needed to be done?
A substitute amoxicillin for metronidazole and prescribe a 2-week course of eradication drugs
B continue omeprazole long-term
C try second-line eradication drugs
D request a ^{13}C urea breath test
E accept matters as they were

34 Which of the following is not true for primary chronic open-angle glaucoma?
A untreated, it gradually leads to tunnel vision
B Afro-Caribbean origin is a risk factor
C acetazolamide should be avoided if the eGFR is 35 ml/minute/1.75m^2 or less
D reduction in the trabecular meshwork drainage impairs the flow of aqueous humour from the ciliary body through the pupil
E the eye is painful and corneal oedema leads to the appearance of haloes around lights

35 Miss Eunice Edith, aged 82 years, joined a new Practice when she moved to live with her elderly sister. She was well and only took two tablets of paracetamol most bedtimes.

Examination: BP 150/88; no abnormal physical signs.

Routine blood test results showed a plasma sodium of 128. Records showed that the electrolyte had been of the same order for the previous 6 years.

What should Miss Edith's new GP do?
A have the assay repeated
B repeat the assay together with paired plasma and spot urine osmolality and sodium measurements
C prescribe desmopressin (DDAVP)
D write a FP10 for demeclocycline
E accept the situation

36 Urinary dipstick testing in a frail 20-year-retired school mistress showed glucose ++, protein ++, nitrites: absent, leucocyte esterase: positive; pH 6.5, specific gravity 1020.

Which of A to E is correct?
A there was pyuria
B a mid-stream urine test (MSU) will grow a coliform
C nitrofurantoin would be a suitable drug
D the patient had renal failure
E the prostatic specific antigen (PSA) is likely to be raised

37 Concerning a fractured neck of femur; which is the odd one out?
A shortening and rotation of the leg is seen in 95% or more of cases
B this fracture does not necessarily prevent walking
C traction is the preferred treatment if there is sarcopenia
D 30-day operative mortality ranges from 15 to 20%
E the signs in 'A' may indicate the presence of a total hip replacement

38 Which one of the following pairs is not strictly an aid to everyday living?
A dressing and grooming
B domestic and leisure
C feeding and bathing
D mood and mentation
E toileting and transfers

39 Nicoladides Makarios left his Limassol restaurants in the hands of his grandsons so as to visit London, his sons and their families. He fell at Trafalgar Square, tore a varicose vein and bled copiously. Blood values noted in a local A & E facility:

Hb	10.2
MCV	70
MCHC	24
RBC count	6.0×10^{12} (4.4–5.8×10^{12}/L)
blood film:	hypochromic, microcytic cells
ferritin	125

What was the explanation of these findings?
A iron deficiency
B B_{12} deficiency
C chronic brucellosis
D thalassaemia major
E thalassaemia trait

40 An 81-year-old otherwise well woman presented with constipation. She took a compound tablet preparation containing calcium and vitamin D four times daily.

Investigations:

sodium	137
potassium	3.9
creatinine	80
calcium	3.0
phosphate	0.8

What was the most likely diagnosis?
A hypercalcaemia due to bony metastases
B hypercalcaemia from bronchogenic carcinoma
C primary hyperparathyroidism
D myeloma
E vitamin D excess

41 Seventy-eight-year-old Irene Felty had painful restricted movements of her hips, ulna deviation of her hands with subluxation of the metacarpophalangeal joints. The proximal interphalangeal joints were in fixed flexion; there was a ruptured extensor tendon.

Which of the following apply?
A the description of the hand is atypical for rheumatoid arthritis
B a raised toilet seat would be helpful
C one would expect Heberden's nodes to be found
D the patient is likely to have the HLA B27 antigen
E a rollator with hand-operated brakes would be of value

42 Winston Manley worked hard from when he arrived in Britain on the MV *Empire Windrush* (1948) in his early 20s. In 2012 his doctor chose to treat his sustained hypertension of 180/115 because of a hypertensive retinopathy. According to the NICE (2011) recommendations, which drug from the following groups should not be prescribed?
A thiazides
B angiotensin II receptor blockers (ARBs)
C calcium channel blockers (CCBs)
D β-blockers
E α-blockers

43 One summer afternoon a practice Sister sampled blood in the home of an elderly bed-bound woman with chronic heart failure. Return to the surgery was delayed by a punctured tyre. The blood samples remained in the Sister's car overnight and were sent to the local hospital laboratory the following morning. At noon results were telephoned to the surgery:

creatinine	130
eGFR	35
K$^+$	6.6

What was the correct action?
A   arrange for an urgent ECG
B   organise prompt transfer to hospital
C   send a prescription for Resonium A
D   ring the patient
E   have a fresh blood sample taken and assayed for K$^+$

44 On the 3rd of November 1906 Herr Prof Dr Alois Alzheimer (1864–1915) presented the clinical and neuropathological findings of his patient Auguste D at a meeting.

Which one of the following is not a feature of the dementia (AD) which has his name?
A   atrophy of temporal and frontal lobes with ventricular dilation
B   the incidence peaks at about 90 years of age
C   the incidence of AD increases exponentially from the sixth decade, doubling every 5 years
D   in becoming hyperphosphorylated, τ (tau) protein changes from a very soluble to a very insoluble compound
E   there is an association between AD and sub-acute bacterial endocarditis

45 On the day of his golden wedding anniversary Derby was admitted to a hyper-acute stroke unit, leaving Joan in their jointly owned £200 000 cottage. Derby had £35 000 savings and a state pension (£120.00 weekly). He did not recover beyond needing a hoist for bed to chair transfers and had to fund his long-term nursing home charges from his savings.

Which of the following statements is correct?
A   all of Derby's £35 000 savings will need to be spent on nursing home fees
B   all of his pension will go towards his residential expenses
C   the cottage will have to be sold to defray nursing home costs
D   £23 250 will be left from Derby's savings
E   Joan will lose her cottage

46 What is the most likely cause of a chronic paronychia in septuagenarians and their elders?
A onycholysis
B diabetes
C malabsorption
D candida infection
E iron deficiency anaemia

47 Which one of the following imaging signs is not red flag material?
A Kerley B line
B apple core
C pepper-pot skull
D honeycomb lung
E two commas

48 Concerning the feet in elderly people; of the following, which is incorrect?
A nails thicken and yet become brittle
B there are insufficient state funded chiropody services
C as age advances many cannot reach their feet
D absent ankle jerks may be of no consequence
E nail pitting suggests combined sub-nutrition and calcium deficiency.

49 Of the various tools available, which is the most appropriate when quantifying a pressure ulcer of a heel in a 78-year-old diabetic man bed-bound because of vascular dementia?
A Waterlow
B Rivermead
C Gleason
D Hamilton
E Barthel

50 Miss Sue Ship, born on 11th November 1918, had a total hip replacement on a Monday. On Thursday, whilst eating porridge, she developed sudden dyspnoea. Drugs: dabigatran 150 mg daily and paracetamol 1 g qds.

Which of the following favoured a pulmonary embolus (PE)?
A a D-dimer of ×3 above the reference range
B a right bundle block
C a normal departmental chest x-ray
D FEV_1/VC ratio of 70%
E oxygen saturation of 80% whilst on 15 L oxygen gas via a non-rebreathing mask

51 At the age of 70 Miss Jean Brody was blinded by glaucoma. Nevertheless, she lived alone very successfully; she learnt Braille, and enjoyed Radio 4 and RNIB talking books. Her guide dog Crème guided her twice-daily walks, twice-weekly visits to a swimming pool and to her social events. After 15 years Crème developed a malignancy and had to be put down. Miss Brody lost the companionship of her dog, her independence, mobility and social life. Her visitors, mainly ex-pupils, saw untouched pre-cooked meals and a subdued, introspective, monosyllabic, shuffling old woman. Physical examination and blood tests were unremarkable.

What was the diagnosis?
A hypothyroidism
B occult malignancy
C dementia
D depression
E social isolation

52 Bleddyn Ieuan Davies was a 'baby boomer' of the Great War. For 51 years he worked in the coal-mining industry of the Rhondda Valleys. He was excused military service in World War II on account of the importance of his job. After retirement, dyspnoea gradually worsened and in his late 70s he repeatedly coughed up black sputum.

What was Mr Davies' industry-related condition?
A lung cancer
B mesothelioma
C progressive massive fibrosis
D coalworker's simple pneumoconiosis
E silicosis

53 Which is correct regarding the Liverpool Care Pathway for the Dying Patient (LCP)?
A once established, the LCP authority lasts either 14 or 21 days
B once on the LCP, a patient's assisted nutrition and hydration are automatic
C the LCP is to meet the dying patient's best interests
D once set up, LCP detail does not need altering
E the Pathway is exclusive to elderly people dying of malignancies

54 A new calcium tablet became available. A group of 300 patients was selected to assess the acceptability of the new preparation. The end point was to find how many of the subjects were taking the preparation 12 months later. Which one of the following study designs is the appropriate tool to answer the study question?

A case-controlled study

B cohort study

C cross-sectional study

D randomised controlled study

E a meta analysis

55 A 77-year-old man was voluntarily admitted to a Medical Assessment Unit. He was unwashed, dishevelled, physically aggressive and verbally abusive. During the night he hit a staff nurse, attempted to strangle himself with infusion tubing after stabbing his neck with a plastic fork and tried to throw himself out of a fifth floor window. Security staff had to restrain him from attempting to leave the Ward 'to end it all'.

Under which section of the mental health legislation was he detained as an informal patient?

A section 13(5)

B section 2(3)

C section 3(2)

D section 5(4)

E section 5(2)

56 The social model of disability assumes which of the following?

A that a person's disability is not the factor causing discrimination

B that the organisation of society discriminates against the disabled

C there is a degree of antagonism between health professionals in disability and the disability liberating movements

D teenagers are unwittingly ageist because they tend to hold and to act as if the ages of 60 years and more are 'over the hill' and unnecessarily consume resources – 'you greedy, pathetic old man'

E the absence of ramps for entry to a public library is a combined attitudinal and architectural statement against physically handicapped individuals

57 80-year-old Mr Ash, a Bristolian who had worked for WD & HO Wills, was dying of lung cancer. Mrs Ash, who has achieved a 52-pack-year history asked for a tablet to 'help me stop'. Which of the following could have been combined with behavioural support therapy?
  A lorezepam
  B bupropion
  C 25 mg nicotine patch
  D citalopram
  E vardenafil

58 KG Pound, born 1931, weighed himself daily under standard conditions and recorded his weight. After 4 months of unchanged weight he gained 5.5 kg over 30 days, developed orthopnoea and New York Heart Failure Class III dyspnoea.

What should he have done?
  A double his daily 25 mg dose of eplerenone
  B double the daily 40 mg dose of furosemide
  C change to bumetanide 1 mg daily
  D restrict his tea intake
  E contact his doctor

59 Starting in 2005 John Bull's days were increasingly painful and frightening. Sleep was punctuated by flashbacks to traumatic battlefield events experienced when a 20-year-old private in the Korean War (1950–53). In order to sleep, he began to drink excessively and because he needed 'to be alone with my memories', he withdrew from family and friends.

What was the probable diagnosis?
  A alcoholism
  B late onset depression
  C post-traumatic stress disorder
  D repeated anxiety attacks
  E bipolar dysfunction

60 Which one of the following abnormal laboratory variables is present in the majority of patients at the time of diagnosis of multiple myeloma?
  A Hb < 10
  B $Ca^{2+} > 2.8$
  C β_2-microglobulin > 5.5
  D urate > 0.5
  E creatinine > 180

61 Regarding Do Not Attempt to Resuscitate (DNAR) decisions; which of the following is correct?

   A the wishes of a competent patient may be overruled by a senior doctor deemed to be deciding in the best interests of the patient

   B the Mental Capacity Act 2005 gives the clinician the authority to override the wishes of a patient with capacity and the relatives

   C over the whole of the NHS the probability of successful resuscitation efforts in a woman over 80 years is about 9%

   D in hospital a DNAR order may be rescinded at any time

   E a valid advanced directive insisting on resuscitation in any or all circumstances may be set aside if common sense indicates that such efforts would be likely to fail.

62 The elderly Mr Hale Hearty had a BMI of 35 kg/m². Liver function tests showed a persistent, isolated elevation of alanine transaminase 2.5 to 3.0 times above the reference range.

   Hepato-biliary ultrasound showed 'bright echoes' from the liver, some stones in the gall bladder and bile ducts of normal dimensions.

   What was the diagnosis?

   A primary biliary cirrhosis

   B intermittent duct obstruction

   C idiopathic cirrhosis

   D non-alcoholic fatty liver disease

   E right heart failure

63 Which of the following is the best way of expressing renal function to make it most comprehensible?

   A as serum creatinine

   B as creatinine clearance (UV/P)

   C by using the Cockroft & Gault equation (CG)

   D by using the chronic kidney disease (CKD) classification

   E by using the modification of diet in renal disease (MDRD) study equation

64 Mr Salt was both depressed and hypertensive. At the first consultation citalopram 10 mg and bendroflumethiazide 2.5 mg were prescribed. Four weeks later he was argumentative, variably confused and said odd things.

Examination: euvolaemic, BP 148/97 lying, 142/92 standing

Investigations:

creatinine	90
sodium	122
potassium	4.3
calcium	2.5
Hb	12.0
TSH	0.9
CRP	11

What needed to be done?
A   ask for psychiatric help
B   stop citalopram
C   stop the thiazide
D   stop both
E   suggest that Mr and Mrs Salt have a holiday together

65 Regarding the mouth in the elderly, which is correct:
A   the edentulous state tends to be social class related
B   salivary flow rates are maintained
C   dentures should be worn overnight
D   most oral malignancies are squamous cell carcinomas
E   there is a natural aversion to invading another person's mouth

66 An 80-year-old chap with well-controlled type II diabetes developed dyspnoea and bilateral pitting oedema to the patellae. He took an angiotensin converting enzyme inhibitor (ACEI) for hypertension and furosemide for congestive heart failure.

Investigations showed:

chest x-ray: features of overload
left ventricular ejection fraction: 50% of reference range
HbA_{1c}: 7.0 (53)

Which one of the following drugs as monotherapy would be the most suitable to avoid additional fluid retention?
A   basal insulin
B   saxagliptin
C   gliclazide
D   pioglitazone
E   diazoxide

67 A 75-year-old woman had a 6-month history of dyspnoea of exertion with swollen ankles at the end of each day. CXR and ECG indicated left ventricular dysfunction. The patient only took occasional paracetamol.

Which pair of drugs needed to be started promptly?
A furosemide and spironolactone
B bendroflumethiazide and spironolactone
C furosemide and perindopril
D perindopril and bendroflumethiazide
E digoxin and furosemide

68 Which one of the syndromes below best fits the following description?
   A grouping of self-neglect, avoiding human contact, living in conditions which become squalid and with a great reluctance to discard used items. There is lack of insight with lack of concern about the person's previous circumstances.
A Charles Bonnet's
B Hallpike
C Ramsay-Hunt
D Diogenes
E Ekbom's

69 An 83-year-old man had progressive dyspnoea for 24 or more months. There were no other features.

Examination: oxygen saturation on air 84%; 'velcro-like' sounds widely heard over lower third of both lungs.

What was the diagnosis?
A pulmonary fibrosis
B congestive heart failure
C multiple pulmonary emboli
D asthma
E COAD

70 Haematemesis led a 74-year-old woman to have an endoscopy. The base of a bleeding gastric ulcer was infiltrated with adrenaline. Two days later she was discharged to her home. In clinic, in three weeks time, she was well.

Which, of the following, was the then best managerial step?
A continue a proton pump inhibitor (PPI) for the foreseeable future
B discharge from hospital follow up
C repeat the OGD six weeks after the original to check ulcer healing and site
D perform a ^{13}C urea breath test to assess *H pylori* infestation
E request *H pylori* serology to confirm success

71 Which one of the following is incorrect?
   A the majority of people over 85 are widows
   B telomere length correlates with longevity
   C viewed historically, ageing is a recent development
   D the majority of physiological changes occurring with increasing age are detrimental
   E the free radical theory of ageing is now discredited

72 Urinary incontinence developed in an 83-year-old man. Urine dipstick testing was positive for nitrites but negative for leukocyte esterase.

   Which of the following was correct?
   A atypical bacterial products reduce nitrites to nitrates
   B coliform bacteria were present
   C if the dipstick was negative for both leucocyte esterase and nitrites, the urine would have been sterile on culture
   D a negative nitrite result would exclude the presence of resistant bacteria
   E a 5-day course of a cephalosporin would be appropriate

73 One December, a 79-year-old man was diagnosed as having Parkinson's disease. By the following June his wife reported that he had developed visual hallucinations, was increasingly forgetful and was unsteady on his feet. 'The tablets don't seem to be working as well as they did at first.'

   Drugs: simvastatin, aspirin, perindopril and co-beneldopa.

   What was the probable diagnosis?
   A Alzheimer's disease
   B cerebrovascular disease
   C levodopa psychosis
   D depression
   E Lewy Body disease

74 Persistent lumbar pain in an 84-year-old woman was found to be due to osteoporotic collapse. She was on no treatment.

   Together with analgesics, what should have been prescribed?
   A calcium tablets
   B cholecalciferol
   C a bisphosphonate
   D calcium tablets with vitamin D
   E bisphosphonate with vitamin D and calcium

75 Poppy and Polly were octogenarian, monovular twin spinsters. For 25 years Poppy had suffered from painful, relentlessly progressive, destructive, crippling rheumatoid arthritis. After much thought and discussion with her sister, Poppy decided that she would travel to Switzerland so as to die at an assisted suicide clinic before she became immobilised by the severity of her nociceptive pain.

Barthel index 7/20; geriatric depression scale 4/15; AMTS 10/10.

Assuming that Poppy remained inflexible in her plan, what was appropriate?
A respect Poppy's decision
B inform both GP and rheumatologist
C consult a pain management physician
D ask a Macmillan nurse to call
E use increasing doses of opiates

76 Concerning benign essential tremor: which one is incorrect?
A improves with taking ethanol
B is often inherited
C the tremor worsens with activity
D affects the arms in about 90% of patients
E constipation is almost universal

77 Mr White had been satisfactorily anticoagulated with warfarin for atrial fibrillation since his 78th birthday. His INR always lay close to the target value of 2.5. At the end of a 5-day course of ampicillin his INR was found to be 7.0. There was no bruising or bleeding.

Which of the following was the best course of action?
A stop warfarin
B stop ampicillin
C stop both and give vitamin K
D stop both and check the INR in 48 hours
E stop both, give vitamin K and infuse clotting factors

78   Five years after the beginning of his old age pension the asymptomatic CM Luke was found to have chronic myeloid leukaemia (CML). His retirement proceeded without difficulty with the CML well controlled by a tyrosine kinase inhibitor. Suddenly he became 'off colour' with evening temperature and sweating, bled more than usual when he nicked himself whilst shaving and bruised easily.

Investigations: wbc 40×10^9/L
                  platelets 15×10^9/L

What had happened?
A   tyrosine kinase toxicity
B   blastic transformation
C   hypersplenism
D   opportunistic marrow infection
E   marrow failure

79   Which of the following is a cardinal feature of idiopathic Parkinson's disease?
A   symmetrical, slow 4–6 Hz tremor at rest
B   early postural instability
C   rigidity eased by use of the contra-lateral limb
D   bradykinesia of muscle movement
E   retropulsion

80   The paramedics found Mr Lionheart on the floor of a Waitrose store. He was thought to have fainted. Medications: aspirin, simvastatin.

Examination: Glasgow Coma Scale 12 (E4, V4, M5); BP 180/90; pulse regular, 22–24 bpm.

Rhythm strip: P-waves regular and independent of regular wide QRS complexes.

Diagnosis?
A   a simple vaso-vagal event
B   sinus bradycardia
C   heart attack
D   bifascicular block
E   third-degree heart block

81 At her 81st birthday party Susan Bodkin suddenly became amnesic with loss of ante- and retrograde memory. She drove home bewildered but fully conscious. Two hours later she was her normal self but had persistent amnesia for the period of the events.

What was the diagnosis?
A complex partial absence seizure
B cataplexy
C transient global amnesia
D transient epileptic amnesia (temporal lobe dysfunction)
E transient ischaemic attack

82 What is the correct order to apply graduated four-layer compression bandaging when:

  wool bandage = 1,
  crepe bandage = 2,
  elasticated bandage = 3 and
  self-adhesive elasticated bandage = 4?

A 2,1,4,3
B 2,3,1,4
C 1,3,2,4
D 1,2,3,4
E 1,2,4,3

83 A 79-year-old retired bus driver with a 50-pack-year smoking history had two bacterial episodes of exacerbation of chronic obstructive pulmonary disease (COPD). Despite stopping cigarettes he was dyspnoeic climbing a flight of stairs and had to use a salbutamol inhaler prn. He asked for help to reduce his chances of further COPD exacerbations.

What is the best drug recommendation assuming his FEV_1 was, at best, 65% of predicted?
A terbutaline
B inhaled corticosteroid
C oral corticosteroid
D a long-acting β_2 agonist (LABA)
E formoterol + inhaled corticosteroid

84 Which one of the following cranial nerves is not involved in mastication and swallowing?
A V
B VI
C IX
D X
E XII

85 For people dying of non-cancerous causes, which is correct?
   A opiate drugs are too risky in terminal COPD cases: respiratory depression being possibly fatal
   B the nausea and vomiting of end-stage heart failure responds well to cyclizine
   C hyperkalaemia is a painful way to die
   D multiple sclerosis almost invariably leads to a pain-free death
   E implanted cardioverter-defibrillators need to be reprogrammed to pacing mode only.

86 For the past month, after a fall, Guy George, aged 75 years, had progressive right-sided weakness. Gayner George, his sister, said that her brother had difficulty in finding the correct words in some contexts and that his thinking speed had slowed.

   Past history: ischaemic heart disease and hypertension diagnosed after a traffic accident 2 months previously.

   Drugs: perindopril, aspirin and simvastatin.

   Examination: speech non-fluent; mild right hemiparesis; no sensory loss.

   What was the diagnosis?
   A left parietal tumour
   B Alzheimer's dementia
   C left parietal meningoma
   D sporadic Creutzfeldt-Jakob disease
   E sub-dural haematoma

87 Mrs Hay had been a Land Girl during the Second World War (1939–45) and married a farmer. In 2005 she gradually developed a 2-cm dark yellow/black plaque which appeared to stand out from the surrounding skin, and stuck on, her right cheek. The lesion was oval with well-defined edges and had a granular surface. It became warty.

   What was the likely diagnosis?
   A seborrhoeic wart
   B actinic keratosis
   C basal cell carcinoma
   D squamous cell carcinoma
   E melanoma

88 At 23.00 hours one Saturday the duty SHO attended an 83-year-old woman who had thrombosed the distal quarter of her left middle cerebral artery. Glasgow Coma Scale (GCS) 6/15 (E1, V2, M3). There was an advanced directive stating that she did not want life-sustaining treatments but in the urgency in getting to hospital it had been left behind. There was no record in the notes. By 12.10 a.m. on the Sunday, while she fulfilled the criteria for thrombolysis, her tearful husband repeatedly said 'let her go, Doc'.

Which of the following was appropriate?
A intubate and infuse recombinant tissue plasminogen activator (rt-PA)
B use a nasogastric tube urgently to give aspirin and statin syrups
C give a therapeutic dose of subcutaneous low molecular weight heparin
D treat the BP of 180/115 with an infusion of labetalol
E phone a friend

89 Alice Slim had community-acquired pneumonia and at the age of 82 had, over the previous 5 weeks of illness, lost about 20% of her body weight. Serum albumin 21 g/L. She was too unwell to adequately feed herself and the ward too poorly staffed to spend 2–3 hours daily feeding her. Relatives had died. A nasogastric tube was passed and a dietician supplied a nutritionally balanced enteral feed, which ran for 20 hours each day. Whilst being fed late one evening Miss Slim had a sudden onset of tachypnoea and cough. Oxygen saturation at a flow rate of 16 L/minute via a non-rebreathing mask was 80%.

What was the likely diagnosis?
A aspiration of feed
B pulmonary embolus
C bronchopneumonia
D recrudescence of original infection
E pneumothorax

90 An 'all the sevens' (77) year-old man was involved in a head-on collision whilst driving to bingo. In A & E he opened his eyes to pain, mumbled incomprehensibly and resisted attempts to gain vascular access.

What was the GCS score for this man?
A 3
B 8
C 10
D 12
E 13

91 Which of the following is not a risk factor for falling in an elderly person?

A the consumption of more than four different medicines daily

B the use of bi-focal spectacles

C a heat wave

D a recliner chair

E early Parkinson's disease

92 A new non-invasive diagnostic test was developed to determine whether a given person had Alzheimer's dementia. The authors claimed that their test approached the 'gold standard' in diagnostic medicine. Did they mean that their test had:

A a very high specificity and sensitivity

B a very high sensitivity but not specificity

C a very high specificity but not sensitivity

D a very high positive predictive value

E a very high negative predictive value

93 During her 77th year, a woman developed an impaired appetite, palpitations, excessive sweating, systemic malaise and neck pain.

Examination: pulse: sinus at 100 bpm; BP 140/75; thyroid very tender

Investigations:

Ca^{2+}	2.55
wbc	10.9
TSH	0.15
cortisol raised 50% above reference range	
thyroid antibodies: strongly positive	

Which of the following was the most suitable drug?

A propranolol

B carbimazole

C radio iodine

D prednisolone

E propylthiouracil

94 In the older person, ranitidine is preferred to cimetidine because

A of its greater bioavailability

B of its reduced enzyme induction propensity

C of the smaller chance of side-effects

D it is easier to swallow

E cimetidine tablets are more costly

95 Mrs Mary England, aged 77 years, developed a very slowly progressive, red, crusting, sharply marginated, eczematous lesion around her left nipple. This solitary lesion did not respond to emollients, potent topical steroids, antibiotic or antifungal creams.

What was the diagnosis?
A eczema vulgaris
B nickel allergy
C peau d'orange
D Paget's disease
E carcinoma en cuirasse

96 Eighty-three-old Mike Foot (T2DM 13 years) attended his local ED because of a recently developed 1-cm ulcer on one of his clawed toes. There was a sensory neuropathy, the pale skin was hairless and the CRT 5 seconds. 'Them new shoes don't 'elp'.

What was the correct step forwards?
A fix an appointment with the multidisciplinary foot team for the next day
B arrange an appointment for the above team within 7–10 days
C take a swab, have routine bloods sampled and request a clinic appointment for an endocrine clinic
D as for C, plus oral metronidazole and flucloxacillin
E admit via Medical Assessment Unit (MAU) for intravenous antibiotics

97 Earl Grey, aged 87 years, was demented (mini-mental 13/30), had developed neurological dysphagia and aspirated fluids. He lived in a nursing home, was unable to walk and did not recognise his wife or children. He did not aspirate when given fluids thickened to a custard consistency but spat out much of the material. His only pleasure was drinking tea, despite some coughing and choking. A number of efforts to insert a nasogastric tube had been resisted strongly, verbally and physically.

Which was the correct management step?
A allow him freely to eat and drink whatever he wants
B refer him to an old age psychiatrist
C arrange for insertion of a percutaneous endoscopic gastrostomy tube
D sedate and insert a nasogastric tube
E set up a subcutaneous infusion of normal saline

98 The 'Get Up and Go' test involves:
A arising from being seated, turning through 360° and sitting again
B arising and walking 10m
C arising, walking 6m then returning to the seat
D arising, walking 10ft, returning to chair and sitting
E arising, walking 6ft, turning and returning to seat

99 Which of the following is not true concerning a delirium?

A altered level of consciousness is common
B the onset is acute
C the degree of delirium fluctuates
D long-term memory is preserved
E cognitive decline progresses gradually

100 For an audit project an SHO decided to study the choice of prescribing different bisphosphonates in 6 different wards in 2 separate hospitals. Which was the appropriate statistical technique that answered the study question?

A cohort study
B case control study
C cross-sectional study
D randomised controlled study
E a meta analysis

101 The following results became available from an 88-year-old stuperose woman brought to the emergency facility of the Hospital Universitario during a prolonged July heat wave in central Madrid. The Policia Municipal had broken into her flat because neighbours had not seen her for 48 hours.

Examination: she responded only to painful stimuli; pulse, sinus 130; BP 85/40; respiratory rate 28; temperature 41° C; oxygen saturation 85% on air.

Blood variables:		
	wbc	23.5
	Hb	17.0
	Na^+	152
	K^+	5.5
	creatinine	350
	glucose	2.1
	albumin	75

What was the diagnosis?

A urinary tract infection
B acute (intrinsic) renal failure/acute kidney injury (ARF/AKI)
C hyperpyrexia
D intracerebral bleed
E community-acquired pneumonia

102 An 82-year-old woman was admitted with easy bruising and spontaneous gum bleeds. She had lived in an isolated state, surviving on tea and toast and not having left her home for 4 years. Medical, nursing and social service help had been refused robustly.

Examination: distorted hyperplastic gums, rotten loose teeth, bruising of legs with perifollicular bleeds over thighs.

Investigation:

Hb	10.1
MCV	84
MCHC	28
thrombin time	20 sec
INR	1.8
APTT	28 sec (26–40)

The INR was corrected with IV vitamin K but not the bruising. What was the most likely cause of the bleeding?
A iron deficiency
B scurvy
C myelosclerosis
D folate deficiency
E myeloma

103 Dr Jim Dale, OBE, retired after 50 years of general practice but his memory deteriorated, he was unsteady on his feet, had falls, became dysarthric and developed a mild tremor.

Examination: gait: wide-based; normal facial movements; BP 134/88; mini-mental state examination (MMSE) 21/30.

A colleague prescribed L dopa, then donepezil and subsequently citalopram but without benefit.

What was the likely diagnosis?
A progressive nuclear palsy
B frontal meningioma
C multi-system atrophy
D Lewy body dementia
E atherosclerotic pseudo-parkinsonism

104 In January 2012, 80-year-old Percy Porcelain had urinary symptoms. At that time his eGFR was 53 ml/minute/1.73 m². He was prescribed tamsulosin 400 mcg nocte daily. Symptoms worsened with increasing nocturia. By Easter 2012 the eGFR was 12. What was the likely explanation for the change in renal function?

A chronic glomerulonephritis

B obstructive uropathy

C essential hypertension

D diabetic nephropathy

E Peyronie's disease

105 A fellow registrar sometimes did not appear for ward rounds and when present tended to be vague and made odd suggestions. You suspected that he was abusing alcohol or some other psychoactive drug.

What had to be done?

A let sleeping dogs lie – he's a good chap

B swap ward rounds and clinics – he was perhaps safer in outpatients

C tell him his behaviour is worrying

D whistle-blow: speak to the directorate medical lead

E continue to cover up; his wife is pregnant with their fourth child.

106 Which is the least gastrotoxic of the non-selective, non-steroidal anti-inflammatory drugs for an elderly person?

A ibuprofen

B diclofenac

C azapropazone

D ketoprofen

E phenylbutazone

107 Concerning occupational therapists, which of the following are applicable?

A are full members of the multi-disciplinary team

B perform access visits with a physiotherapist, social worker or care manager

C home visits are only performed while the patient is in a ward

D provide aids and devices to help patients regain independent lives

E help by supplying domestic sensory aids

108 Which of the following about tuberculosis (TB) is incorrect?

A the Mantoux test becomes positive in post-primary TB infection

B lifelong immunity to re-infection results from well-treated pulmonary TB in elderly patients

C erythema nodosum may be a presenting feature of TB infection

D TB bacilli are acid and alcohol fast

E the bacilli usually lodge in lung apices

109 Which of the following cranial nerves is wrongly paired with its contribution to swallowing?
 A trigeminal: muscles of mastication and sensation to the anterior two thirds of the tongue and oral cavity.
 B facial: innervation of orbicularis oris (lip closure) and sensation and taste to the posterior one third of the tongue.
 C glossopharyngeal: gag and cough reflexes, sensory innervations of tonsils, laryngeal mucosa and soft palate.
 D vagus: phonation, vocal cord closure. Sensory and motor fibres to oesophagus.
 E hypoglossal: tongue movements.

110 An 82-year-old woman had an embolic stroke. She made a good recovery, becoming fully independent, but remained incontinent. MMSE: 28/30. Her diabetic and varicose ulcers healed, her atrial fibrillation was well controlled and anticoagulation with warfarin easy to maintain. Her pre-admission Barthel index was 20 and at discharge, 18.

What feature explained the change in the index?
 A atrial fibrillation
 B diabetes
 C the ulcer diathesis
 D incontinence
 E the stroke history

111 Barry H____ began to make entirely proper but, for his age (76), excessive sexual demands of his wife. Over the next 6 months he was often seen in the red light district of his town, patronising sex shops and running up a substantial bill on sex phone lines. Well-thumbed 'girly' magazines were found in his den. He was arrested for exposing himself in a children's ward.

What was the most likely explanation?
 A normal pressure hydrocephalus
 B fronto-temporal dementia
 C B_{12} deficiency
 D neurosyphilis
 E Parkinson's disease

112 After a debilitating pneumonia, the previously independent David Clegg (aged 79) began to regain the ability to walk.

Of the various supports available, which allowed the most physiological progress?

A two physiotherapists
B Zimmer frame
C rollator
D delta rollator
E gutter frame

113 Septuagenarian Alfred Thomas had progressive dyspnoea over 2 months.

chest x-ray:	bilateral symmetrical pleural effusions
pleural fluid:	appeared pale yellow
pH	7.45
protein	18.0 g/L
LDH	155 u/L (230–460)
glucose	4.5
micro:	mesothelial cells
culture:	sterile

What was the diagnosis?

A heart failure
B tuberculosis
C empyaemia
D rheumatoid disease
E lung cancer

114 In hypermetropia, which is true?

A the eyeball is too short
B the eyeball is too long
C light focuses in front of the retina
D the cornea has an extra-steep curvature
E the defect can be corrected by a concave lens

115 Over a seven-year period staff of the academic Department of Gerontology at the University Hospital of the Eastern Isles of Scotland conducted a study comparing four-layer compression bandaging of the leg with the usual district nurse care. Eventually 75 patients in each group completed a year's treatment. Results showed that the compression bandaging group had gained an advantage in healing rates compared with the control group. $P < 0.05$.

Which of the following statements was incorrect?
A the result means that the null hypothesis is true
B the result means that the null hypothesis is false
C a 'not significant' result means that there was insufficient evidence of benefit of one ulcer management strategy over the other
D the P value represents the strength of evidence in support of the null hypothesis
E if in a research study $P > 0.05$ the chance of publication is reduced

116 Sandeep Kumar (DOB 1932) gradually developed progressive dyspnoea of exertion, loss of energy and a swollen belly. A CT of chest and abdomen showed distended, overfilled pulmonary and hepatic veins, a normal-sized heart, a calcified pericardium and tense ascites. Ascitic fluid contained a few mesothelial cells, had a protein content of $16\,g/L$ and was sterile on culture.

What was the probable diagnosis?
A occult intra-abdominal malignancy
B asbestosis
C cirrhosis
D TB peritonitis
E constrictive pericarditis

117 What must an elderly person be able to do as part of a mental capacity assessment?
A have a Barthel index of at least 16
B correctly state day, month, year, and name of the deputy prime minister
C use and consider information so as to make a decision
D be able to sign the document of sale
E discuss the decision to be made with the ward sister and registrar

118 An 80-year-old man developed an acutely painful swollen wrist joint.

Investigations:

blood:	urate	345
	wbc	16×10^9L
	CRP	172
	Ca^{2+}	2.38
joint:	fluid:	opalescent yellow
	wbc	$10,000 \times 10^9$/L
	micro:	neutrophils and crystals showing positive birefringence
	culture	sterile
	x-ray:	calcified articular cartilage

What was the diagnosis?
A gout
B pseudogout
C menisical damage
D foreign body in joint
E septic arthritis

119 Dr PD Bradey developed idiopathic Parkinson's disease (PD) at the age of 75 years. His adopted son rang from Gibraltar to enquire of his chances of developing PD.

Which of the following statements was most pertinent during the telephone conversation?
A with an ageing population the number of cases of PD is expected, progressively, to increase
B the incidence of PD lies between 5 and 20/100,000 of the British population
C the prevalence of PD in UK-based studies varies from 110 to 160/100 000
D the onset of PD in the elderly is sporadic
E about 2% of the population aged > 65 years have PD

120 Concerning the use of morphia in people aged 75 years or more, which is correct?
A renal failure is a contraindication
B all patients should receive concomitant lactulose
C morphia analgesia should only be used for cancer-related nociceptive pain
D in the majority of patients there is nausea and vomiting
E almost all patients develop a dry mouth

121 Which of the following is held not to raise the serum concentration of prostate-specific antigen (PSA)?

A ejaculation of semen

B digital prostate examination

C lower urinary tract infection

D horse and bicycle riding

E bladder catheterisation

122 Edith Small was worried when she received a copy of her clinic visit letter in which she was described as 'sarcopenic'. Which of A to E is a description of 'sarcopenia'?

A reduced or lost ankle tendon jerks

B loss of skeletal muscle mass and strength

C bilaterally reduced hand grip

D a 35-second result for the 'Get up and go test'.

E a slow gait

123 Which of the following x-ray report phrases would lead to a referral to a gastrointestinal unit?

A bamboo spine

B Looser's zone

C coin lesion

D omental cake

E azygos lobe

124 An 83-year-old brought her 107-year-old mother to a one stop elderly care outpatient clinic. Over the past three months the mother's shopping had become restricted because of dyspnoea.

Examination: mild pitting oedema; clear chest; BP 135/80; PFR 210 L/minute.

Investigations:

Hb	11.3
creatinine	101
albumin	35
TSH	0.5
BNP	2300 pg/ml (≤ 400)
CRP	8
CXR & ECG:	both normal

What was the probable diagnosis?
A renal failure
B age-related asthma
C sarcopenia
D heart failure
E frailty

125 Mrs G Stone, born on the Armistice Day of the Great War, became delirious, febrile and dehydrated. She was sent from her nursing home to a MAU.

Examination: sarcopenia; sinus rhythm, rate 125; BP 100/65; no localising signs.

Investigations:

urine dip:	negative
CXR:	normal
Hb	10.2
wbc	19.3 with 85% neutrophils
CRP	187
AP	405
ALT	128
bilirubin	35
albumin	32
ferritin	355
blood culture:	gram negative bacteria

What was the likely diagnosis?
A acute cholecystitis
B acute hepatitis
C right basal pneumonia
D portal pyaemia
E secondary liver cancer

126 The day after the 15th birthday party for her transplant kidney, Mrs Graft had a recurrence of her crystal proven gout. She sent her great-granddaughter for a prescription. Her long-term medications: azathioprine, cyclosporine, aspirin, perindopril, statin, omeprazole and zopiclone.

What would not have been a suitable drug for Mrs Graft?
A colchicine
B colchicine with ibuprofen
C allopurinol
D high dose aspirin (> 3 g daily)
E probenecid with urinary alkalisation

127 A 75-year-old man in good health was diagnosed as having T2DM and began appropriate medical management. As months passed, medical restrictions became irksome and were set aside. At 80 he needed a hernia repair. Mid-morning pre-operative blood results:

Hb	11.4
MCV	87
glucose	5.8
HbA$_{1c}$	5.9 (37)
urine pH:	6.2
albumin:creatinine ratio:	22.0 mg/mmol

How were those figures explained?
A the patient restarted his diet and metformin a few days before admission for herniorraphy
B he regained glycaemic control
C he had never lost glycaemic control
D the BM (blood monitoring test strips) under-read the capillary blood glucose concentration
E the laboratory muddled the blood samples

128 Olive Lloyds, an octogenarian, grieved excessively for her husband who had died 5 years previously. She had set her heart on gaining admission to Homley Hall, a well-regarded residential home, but had been turned down. Two old school friends resided there and Olive very much hoped to join them. Otherwise 'there is no point in going on'. Insisting on strict confidence, she told her doctor that if her application was rejected again she had a suitable stock of pills tucked away so that she could use them to 'join John'.

What should her GP have done?
A ring the nursing home to add his weight
B contact a bereavement facility on her behalf
C try to talk her out of it
D prescribe a SSRI or SNRI
E tell Mrs Lloyds' neighbours the circumstances so that they could check her daily

129 Postural hypotension: which of the following is incorrect?
A a fall in SBP ≥ 20 mm Hg on standing from lying
B a fall in DBP ≥ 10 mm Hg from lying to standing
C often occurs with autonomic failure
D found in about 10% of institutionalised people
E not a feature of dehydration

130 'I have always treated angina in 70-year-olds my way and do not need any fancy research to prove me right,' stated the elderly, opinionated, dogmatic Dr T Rex.

Which, from the following hierarchy of evidence would provide the strongest conclusions to support or contradict Dr 'Dinosaur's' belief?
A a cross-sectional survey of patients with angina
B a case-controlled study
C a cohort study
D randomised controlled trials
E meta-analyses

131 Which are indications for long-term oxygen therapy for COPD patients?
A $FEV_1 > 50\%$ of predicted
B oxymetry: saturation – SaO_2 94% (9.3 kPa)
C $PaO_2 < 7.3$ kPa at discharge from hospital with 'clean' lungs
D $PaO_2 < 7.3$ six weeks after resolution of an acute exacerbation
E $PaCO_2$ 6.0–8.5 kPa on air

132 A long-standing tremor worsened during Sam Smith's mid-70s. Mrs Smith feared he was developing Parkinson's disease.

Which of the following made the diagnosis of essential tremor less likely?
A a bilateral symmetrical tremor
B arm and head tremors
C no dysdiadochokinesia
D bradykinesia
E white matter changes on CT brain scan

133 Flo Waters, born 11/11/1918, a resident of a Nursing Home, needed a long-term bladder catheter on account of a mixture of anti-muscarinic unresponsive frequency, urinary incontinence and stress incontinence symptoms.

Which of the following was incorrect?
A she was three times more likely to die during the next year than her non-catheterised fellow residents
B there was a risk of nosocomial infections
C after antibiotics urine testing will be negative
D urethral necrosis may occur
E haematuria may be seen

134 Regarding the toes of elderly patients: which of the following is incorrect?
A   there is fibro-fatty tissue on the plantar aspect of joints
B   clawed toes have deformities of both their intraphalangeal joints
C   hammer toes show fixed flexion of metatarsophalangeal joints
D   hallus valgus stems from lifelong poor gait and inadequate shoe fitting
E   fungal infection between toes is common

135 The stoical Roy Body had put up with a persistent and worsening 'bad back' for decades. When, aged 75 years, he found he was dyspnoeic because he could not take deep breaths, he obtained medical advice. Examination showed an inability to bend his back, his neck was flexed and fixed, chest expansion 1 cm and there was a uveitis. Spine x-ray suggested that human leukocyte antigen B27 should be present: it was.

What was the diagnosis?
A   extensive osteoporosis
B   ankylosing spondylitis
C   sacro-spinal musculo-dystrophy
D   spinal osteochondritis dissecans
E   burnt out juvenile chronic polyarthritis

136 The Very Reverend Emeritus Professor Broughton, born in 1933, had a brain stem stroke which left him with sound thinking but with aphasia, ataxia and unsafe swallowing. He would not accept any form of enteral or parenteral feeding. He scored very highly on non-verbal tests of mental capacity and occupied himself by reading the New Testament in the original Greek. Barthel index 12/20. Serum albumin 22 g/L.

What was the correct management?
A   ask for psychogeriatric help
B   try arguing for the insertion of a nasogastric tube
C   allow the Reverend to have his favourite night cap of a malt whisky and PRN fluids by day
D   sedate him before sending him off for percutaneous endoscopic gastrostomy insertion
E   discuss matters at the weekly Multidisciplinary Team Coordinator (MDT) meeting

137 Nellie Trunk was renowned for her memory and recall. Previously Opposition spokespersons had been trounced at the circus of Prime Minister's questions. In July 2012 she realised that her recall of names and events over the the previous three months had become unreliable. Addenbrooke's Cambridge Examination – Revised (2005): 83/100. Points were lost on anterograde and recall memories.

Which of the memory systems in this 68-year-old woman were failing?
A declarative semantic memory
B declarative episodic memory
C immediate memory
D working memory
E procedural memory

138 What is the most appropriate maintenance dose of digoxin for an incapacitated 80-year-old-year-old woman with atrial fibrillation (AF) and biventricular failure? Other medication: furosemide 40 mg, eplerenone 25 mg and warfarin. All digoxin doses in micrograms of active drug. Body weight 50 kg; eGFR 45 ml/minute/1.73 m².
A one 62.5 daily dose
B a 62.5 dose × 5 days each week
C one 125 tablet alternate days
D one 250 tablet daily
E half a 125 tablet daily

139 John Thomas had pulmonary TB as an undergraduate. He was a lifelong non-smoker. In his mid-70s, whilst receiving chemotherapy for myeloma, he had a haemoptysis.

Chest x-ray: 2 cm cavity in right upper lobe.

Bronchoscopy: refused

What simple, economical test established the diagnosis of reactivation of TB?
A Mantoux skin test
B CT upper half of lungs
C auramine phenol staining and then Ziehl-Neelson staining and Lowestein Jenson (ZN stain & LJ) culture of sputum for Mycobacterium tuberculosis (MTB)
D interferon γ tests (IFNγ)
E gastric washings to capture MTB

140 A 75-year-old chap attends his practice surgery because of low mood, hopelessness and 6 kg weight loss since he had a middle cerebral artery territory stroke 2 months previously. His wife added that her husband often felt that now there was no point in living.

Medical history: T2DM, hypertension and an episode of depression 4 years previously.

Examination: residual hemiparesis, flat affect, tearful with negative thoughts. There was difficulty in maintaining concentration; short-term recall was impaired.

The way forward was?

A a CT scan of the brain to show that there was nothing new to concern doctor or patient

B the cognitive impairment was very suggestive of a co-morbid dementia

C to prescribe at least 6 months of citalopram or other SSRI

D the infarct site was a relevant factor in the development of the affective disturbance

E cognitive behavioural therapy as the principal therapy

141 Concerning Mrs V Ample (DOB 13/01/1934):

Examination: acanthosis nigricans, BMI $38 \, kg/m^2$, basal diastolic pressure 115 mm Hg

Average data obtained over the previous 6 months:

fasting trigylcerides	4.5 (≥ 1.7 mmol/L)
HbA$_{1c}$	9.5 (80)
γGT	250
ALT	190
ACR:	85 mg/mmol
ECG:	LVH and an old inferior transmural infarct
ultrasound imaging of solid abdominal viscera: diffuse fatty infiltration of liver, a few gallstones, bile ducts of normal dimensions.	

The best interpretation of the data was:

A ischaemic heart disease

B severe obesity

C non-alcoholic fatty liver disease (NAFLD)

D type II diabetes mellitus

E metabolic syndrome

142 Worldwide life expectation continues to increase as do the number of centenarians. Which factors do not influence ageing trends?
  A malarial control programs
  B increasing numbers of those with freely disposable 'grey' incomes
  C the post-World War II 'baby boomers'
  D reduction in nicotine addiction
  E improved perinatal medical expertise

143 Which of the following naturally decline with ageing?
  A FEV_1
  B glomerular filtration rate
  C gastric H^+ secretion
  D parathyroid hormone (PTH) secretion
  E cardiac output

144 Regarding eye changes in old age, which of the following is wrong?
  A sunken – due to a reduction in periorbital fat
  B papillary responses to light and accommodation are slowed
  C arcus cornealis – which correlates with cardiovascular disease
  D shortening of the axial length of the eye
  E entropion and ectropion are common

145 Which of the following diminishes the chance of an aspiration pneumonia?
  A good oral care
  B absence of teeth or dentures
  C recurrent laryngeal nerve lesions
  D untreated gastro-oesophageal reflux
  E weakness of the X cranial nerve

146 Which of the following carries neutral weight in respect of falls causation?
  A born before 1945
  B wearing bifocal spectacles
  C calcium channel blocker drugs
  D wet leaves
  E hip/femoral neck protector garments

147 A very spry man born in the late-1930s presented with arthritis, conjunctivitis and diarrhoea after a 10-day holiday at a Thailand tourist resort.

  Which of the following had priority?
  A taking a sexual history
  B advising careful hand washing after elimination
  C booking an appointment with a HIV advisor
  D checking for chlamydia and gonorrhoea
  E referral to a sexual health (VD, GUM) clinic

148 Of the following, which is the least satisfactory opioid choice as an alternative to morphia?

A oxycodone
B methadone
C fentanyl
D buprenorphine
E pethidine

149 Louise Perks was looking peaky. She was cold and tired and could not remember her hectic nursing work during the London Blitz (1940–42). Her indigestion worsened and she stopped her regular tablets (simvastatin, ranitidine, aspirin, atenolol). Physical examination did not help diagnostically.

Blood test results:	Hb	10.0
	MCV	76
	CRP	22
	Na$^+$	134
	K$^+$	haemolysed
	urea	19.8
	creatinine	77
	bilirubin	28
	albumin	38

What was the diagnosis?

A hyponatraemia
B megaloblastic anaemia
C iron deficiency
D malnutrition
E bone marrow dysfunction

150 Iuean Wynn Jones (DOB January 1923) became asthmatic in winter 2009/10. In 2012 he had two pneumonic bouts with additional wheezing. Both events failed adequately to respond to antibiotics and salbutamol.

Investigations:

FEV$_1$	< 50% of predicted
wbc	17.5 with 15% mature eosinophils
CRP	79
IgE	> 1000 mg/ml
IgE RAST	very strongly positive
CXR	collapse/consolidation with proximal bronchiectasis

What was the most likely diagnosis?
A Legionnaire's disease
B allergic broncho-pulmonary aspergillosis
C *Klebsiella pneumoniae* infection
D pulmonary tuberculosis
E idiopathic pulmonary fibrosis

151 A 83-year-old woman had severe morning headaches for a month. She had had classical migraine which stopped around the age of 50 years, and a neck whiplash injury 10 years previously.

What was the most likely cause of her headaches?
A a cerebral tumour
B cranial arteritis
C recurrence of her migraine
D cervical spondylitis
E *Herpes zoster* infection of the 1st division of the V cranial (trigeminal) nerve

152 What was the single most appropriate investigation for a 79-year-old retired civil servant who mentioned to his GP that there was something wrong with his 'old boy'?

Examination: inflamed tip of penis with no discharge. PR: prostate moderately enlarged.
A assay of random plasma glucose
B assay of fasting plasma glucose
C assay of PSA
D assay of glycosylated haemoglobin
E urine dip and MSU

153 An 85-year-old couple spent a warm economical February in a hotel in the Balearic Isles. Upon return to Kent the wife developed a dry cough.

Investigations:

urine:	proteinuria ++, blood +, negative for leucocyte esterase and nitrites
CXR	an inflammatory area in the left lower zone
CRP	45
wbc	10.0
Hb	13.9
Na$^+$	125
K$^+$	4.8

What was the likely diagnosis?
A *Legionella pneumophila* infection
B lobar pneumonia
C broncho-pulmonary aspergillosis
D a pulmonary embolism
E bronchopneumonia

154 Regarding the treatment of a new onset angina in a normotensive non-diabetic, non-smoking man of 75 years. After explaining the use of a nitrate spray, what according to the 2011 NICE recommendations is the first drug to select? Choose from one of the either/or A to E pairs.
A CCB/βB
B nitrate/nicorandil
C simvastatin/fibrate
D ACEI/ARB
E ivabradine/ranotazine

155 Which of the following is the strongest risk factor for stroke at the age of 80 years?
A a BMI = 34 kg/m^2
B hypercholesterolaemia
C cigarette smoking
D diabetes mellitus
E hypertension

156 Regarding leg ulcers: which of the following is correct?
A the majority lie over the course of the long saphenous vein
B the ulcerated leg should not be raised above the level of the right atrium
C lipodermatosclerosis occurs with long-term arterial insufficiency
D chronic venous ulcers become 'punched out' and deep
E the ankle-brachial pressure index (APBI) has a reference range of 0.6 to 1.0

157 Which of the following is not a cardinal feature of Parkinson's disease?
A postural instability
B rest tremor
C bradykinesia
D apathy
E rigidity

158 An 89-year-old woman had increasing fatigue, lethargy and easy sleeping. There were no other features. She had been hypertensive; amlodipine and simvastatin had been stopped 3 years previously because of her age.

Examination: BMI 25 kg/m²; BP 145/95; pulse: sinus rhythm; normal heart sounds; bi-basal crepitations; trivial ankle oedema.

What was the most likely diagnosis?
A chest infection
B recurrent PE
C congestive failure
D late onset asthma
E hypothyroidism

159 Richard Bright, born in the mid-1930s, found that his urine frothed in the toilet pan, his weight went up 'a couple of stone' and his legs became swollen such that only extra-sized slippers would fit.

Investigations:

albumin	27
cholesterol	12.5
urine protein:creatinine ratio:	>350 mg/mmol
ECG & CXR:	normal

What was the diagnosis?
A congestive heart failure
B advanced liver disease
C nephrotic syndrome
D CKD stage 3Ap
E non-alcoholic fatty liver disease

160 Dan Archer, a livestock farmer, played Saturday football to his late 60s when meniscal tears ended his sporting days. Ten years later, whilst herding cows, one of his usually aching knees became very painful and later tensely swollen.

Joint fluid: opalescent yellow with low viscosity
wbc: $15,000 \times 10^9$/L
Culture: awaited

What was the diagnosis?
A   further meniscal damage
B   osteoarthritis (OA)
C   pseudo gout
D   septic arthritis
E   'farmers' arthritis

161 From a 77-year-old man:
1   drenching night sweats
2   AP 429 of hepatic origin; γGT 268 (10–78); microsomal antibodies not detected; Hb 11.4; MCV 92; CRP 327; ESR 111
3   CXR and abdominal ultrasound: no abnormalities found

What was the likely diagnosis?
A   partial intrahepatic bile duct obstruction
B   Wilson's disease
C   primary biliary cirrhosis
D   lymphoma
E   hepatic abscess

162 The Disposable Soma Theory of ageing (DST) states that ageing is caused by accumulation of random tissue damage which is balanced by repair. Repair is metabolically expensive and the amount an organism has available is proportional to its lifespan. Repair may be directed to the organism's soma or its reproductive structures. Logically reproductive potential is more species beneficial than longevity (disposable soma).

Which of the following does the DST not imply or indicate?
A   with unlimited food, immortality would be gained
B   explains why women live longer than men
C   moderate calorie restriction threatens species survival
D   long-lived species will have more offspring
E   the evolutionary value of additional life declines after the age at which the organism gains reproductive maturity

163 At the age of 75 years Dr HT Mann had a right middle cerebral artery ischaemic attack. He was found to be persistently hypertensive. What approximate number of patients are needed to be treated (NNT) to prevent a further CVA at one year?

A 8000

B 50

C 13 000

D 400

E 180

164 Miss Iris Argyle, aged 80, woke to find that she had pain and 'blindness' in one eye.

Examination: upon mechanically lifting the drooping eyelid, the pupil was fixed dilated with the eye turned out and slightly down ('down and out' position).

What was the diagnosis?

A Horner's syndrome

B III cranial nerve palsy

C Holmes-Aide pupil

D ocular myasthenia

E myotonic pupil

165 At 70 Sid Perks' COAD symptoms were much helped by tiotropium and a long-acting β_2-agonist. Five years on, his dyspnoea worsened considerably over a weekend and was unresponsive to rescue salbutamol. His face felt 'full'.

Examination: non-pitting plethoric swelling of face and neck. Non-pulsatile jugular venous pressure (JVP) raised to angle of jaw. Dilated superficial veins over upper arms. BP 120/80; pulse 120, SR; normal heart sounds.

What was the diagnosis?

A right heart failure

B biventricular failure

C constrictive pericarditis

D exacerbation of COAD

E superior vena cava obstruction

166 Mrs Driscoll complained of a 'lump on my eyelid'. Which of the following is an unlikely explanation in an octogenarian?

A chalazion

B stye

C marginal cyst

D molluscum contagiosum

E xanthelasma

167 Miss Snow White was taken to her general practitioner because she had excessive daytime sleepiness despite reasonable nights of sleep.

Which of the following was a likely explanation?
A heart failure
B early dementia
C obstructive sleep apnoea
D restless legs
E hypothyroidism

168 The 95-year-old diminutive, demented, incontinent Edith Sparrow was found to have a linear bruise across her left breast. There was no history of trauma. Over the previous 17 years she had been cared for exclusively by her unmarried daughter, now aged 77 years. Blood tests and bone x-rays were normal. MMSE 13/30. Physical abuse was considered.

Which of the following is incorrect?
A there is an established framework through which suspected cases of abuse may be investigated
B abuse is considered to occur most frequently in the abused person's home
C If possible, the stressed relative who is the abuser should be relieved by respite help, provision of carers and financial help whilst keeping the abused in their usual environment
D poor hygiene, bed sores and malnutrition may represent abuse by neglect
E ageism is a form of elder abuse

169 Which one of the following is incorrect?
A a fasting plasma venous glucose ≥ 7.0 is diagnostic of diabetes mellitus
B a plasma glucose concentration at 2 hours after an oral glucose tolerance test (OGTT) ≥ 11.1 is diagnostic
C impaired glucose tolerance (IGT) comprises a fasting venous glucose of < 7.0 and a 2-hour OGTT of ≥ 11.1
D the definition of impaired fasting glucose involves a venous glucose of ≥ 6.1 and ≤ 6.9 and a 2-hour OGTT venous plasma glucose of < 7.8
E the HbA_{1c} assay is not yet used by WHO for defining various degrees of loss of glycaemic control

170 Which one of the following factors mitigates against polypharmacy (as defined as the use of ≥ 4 drugs daily)?
A multiple active pathologies
B attendance at a number of specialist clinics
C patient expectations of a prescription at each surgery visit
D lack of regular critical review of all medicines
E 'correct use of FP10s help clear the waiting room'

171 Which of the following 5 cranial nerves supplies fibres close the larynx when swallowing?

A V

B VII

C IX

D X

E XII

172 Septuagenarian JT Dolor was carried into A & E on account of a swollen, hot, very painful right knee.

Joint fluid:	appearance:	opaque yellow-green
	wbc	88×10^9/L
	stain:	gram-positive organisms

Before culture results, antibiotics were started. What was the most likely bacterium to be grown?

A *Staphylococcus aureus*

B *Neisseriae meningitidis*

C *Haemophilus influenzae*

D *Streptococcus viridans*

E *Neisseriae gonorrhoea*

173 Drs Fred Goodworks and Jim Welldone were partners before qualifying in 1957. They retired aged 65 years and spent the next 10 years in voluntary medical service in rural tropical Africa. Upon return to England, Fred developed perineal pain, dysuria and frequency. Sterile pyuria was found. Jim organised the following:

> ultrasound of renal tract: nothing abnormal imaged
> metabolic screen for urinary stone: negative
> urine culture for alcohol-acid-fast bacilli (AAFB): no growth at 10 weeks

Diagnosis was made at cystoscopy and was?

A bladder stone

B transitional cell carcinoma

C renal TB

D fastidious organism infection

E schistosomiasis

174 John Fry, aged 83 years, had had gout for the past 5 years and took allopurinol 100 mg daily. He developed an acute attack in his left knee.

Investigations:

Hb	9.9
CRP	55
urate	280
eGFR	30

What was the correct treatment?
A add diclofenac
B substitute diclofenac for allopurinol
C increase allopurinol
D prescribe colchicine
E exchange allopurinol for colchicine

175 Emeritus Prof Gerry Cor collapsed during a mid-December service celebrating his 55 years of association with his College. To avoid fuss he had ignored his worsening symptoms of chest pain, syncope and dyspnoea. He was taken by ambulance from the College chapel to the local ED. A medical registrar noted the following signs: small volume pulse with a slow up stroke; a single 2nd heart sound and a crescendo-decrescendo systolic murmur at the 2nd right intercostal space. BP 140/102.

ECG: R in V_6 plus an S wave in V_1 > 35 mm.

What was Prof Cor's likely diagnosis and outlook?
A mitral regurgitation with risk of thrombo-embolism – begin low molecular weight heparin and warfarin
B mild aortic stenosis – for routine cardiac clinic appointment in January/February next
C critical aortic stenosis – admit for detailed study
D prescribe diuretics with a long-acting nitrate via TTOs to cover the period until a geriatric outpatient clinic in the new year
E complete a HP10 for aspirin, statin, ACEI and a PPI before an outpatient appointment in the new year

176 Eighty-year-old Clive Thomas had become sluggish and constipated, and his declarative episodic and working memories had declined.

Examination gave no clues. MMSE 25/30.

Blood test results:	eGFR	50
	Na$^+$	122
	K$^+$	4.1
	Ca^{2+}	2.3

Which of the following drugs was most likely to have induced this state?
A warfarin sodium
B sodium fusidate
C perindopril
D venlafaxine
E sodium valproate

177 Jim James, aged 81, had a transthoracic replacement of his stenotic aortic valve. Post-operatively oliguric renal failure with infection impaired nutritional intake for 3 weeks. He was too frail to swallow so a nasogastric tube was passed and iso-osmolar enteral nutrition begun.

What was the most likely plasma biochemical finding during the second day of feeding?
A hypercalcaemia
B hyperkalaemia
C hypoglycaemia
D hypocalcaemia
E hypophosphataemia

178 Eighty-four-year-old TC Davies was 'getting on'. He had a Gleason score of 6 calculated from the morphology of his prostatic tissue (carcinoma of prostate range 6–8). Prostate specific antigen 13 mg/ml (cut off 7.2). There was no evidence of metastatic disease.

What was the most appropriate choice for 'TC'?
A castration
B radical prostatectomy
C radical radiotherapy
D cyproterone
E observation

179 Helen Lar (born in the early 1930s) repeatedly attended her general practitioner's surgery because of headaches. She thought she had a cerebral tumour and wanted a 'scan'. There were no physical signs. Her GP reassured her: a brain CT showed modest involutional changes only. A week later Miss Lar returned to ask for a different scan 'in case something had been missed'.

What was the situation?
A   hypochondriasis
B   a non-somatoform disorder
C   an MRI scan will reassure her
D   antidepressants are not indicated
E   repeated reassurance should carry the day, thereby reducing her fears

180 An 81-year-old man was treated with a cephalosporin for a nitrite positive urine dip. A week later he was passing 7 to 8 stage 6 to 7 Bristol stool classification motions each 24 hours. There was no fever or vomiting, nor had there been constipation.

Examination: soft, non-distended, non-tender belly; very offensive green stools.

Blood test results:	Hb	11.7
	wbc	14.0 with 85% neutrophils
	albumin	32
	CRP	55

What was the next investigation?
A   ultrasound of renal tract
B   arrange for a sigmoidoscopy
C   AXR for renal stones
D   ask for colonic endoscopy
E   ask for stool assay for CD toxin

181 Which one of the following questions is not one from the CAGE questionnaire for alcohol misuse?
A   have you recently craved alcohol?
B   has anyone felt you should cut down on your drinking?
C   have you been annoyed by people criticising your drinking?
D   have you ever felt guilty about your drinking?
E   do you need a drink first thing in the morning (eye opener) to get rid of a hangover or steady your nerves?

182 A 79-year-old man who had smoked since he was 18 lost about 10 kg body weight over 3 months.

Biochemical results:	K^+	4.0
	Na^+	122
	creatinine	80
	serum osmolality	249 (275–295 mOsmol/kg)
	urine osmolality	280 (50–800)
	urine sodium	65 (10–150)

What was the diagnosis?

A lung cancer

B syndrome of inappropriate antidiuretic secretion

C renal calculi

D functional polydypsia

E Conn's syndrome

183 Regarding Do Not Attempt to Resuscitate (DNAR) decisions, which are incorrect?

A relatives have the legal right to insist on or reject resuscitation or a DNAR order

B the competent patient may insist that every effort is made to resuscitate him/her against medical opinion

C DNAR decisions do not necessarily require a discussion with the patient

D it is always sensible to take account of the nursing staff's opinions when considering setting up a DNAR order

E it is very unlikely for resuscitation to re-establish respiration and circulation in a patient who, pre-arrest, had left ventricular failure with hypotension

184 Side-effects of antidepressant drugs include:

A vomiting

B diarrhoea

C gastritis and duodenal ulceration

D hallucinations

E neuroleptic malignant syndrome

185 An 88-year-old widow attended her neighbourhood A & E. She was the sole carer for her 64-year-old son with cerebral palsy. He could not dress or mobilise without her help. The mother, while fully compos mentis, had been unable to walk for the past 48 hours and was distressed because her condition prevented her from helping her son.

Urine dip: positive for leucocyte esterase

What was the best choice for mother and son?
A arrange for carers to visit four times daily to help the son
B arrange for both to be admitted to a residential home
C arrange for both to be admitted to the local A & E ward
D arrange for the son to be admitted into respite care
E arrange for the mother to receive nitrofurantoin BD

186 What is the commonest cause of erectile dysfunction in men in their late 70s?
A psychological – fear of failure
B hypogonadism
C disinterest
D diabetes
E α-blockade

187 One Sunday afternoon whilst making a cake, 89-year-old Mrs Sam Prescott took a heavy fall, fracturing a wrist and pubic rami. She was found on Monday morning on her kitchen floor. On Tuesday her small volume of urine was a deep red/brown colour ('coca cola' urine).

What measurement would make the diagnosis?
A serum creatinine
B urine dip for leucocyte esterase and nitrites
C urine microscopy
D blood or urine for myoglobin assay
E paired blood and urine samples for Na^+ assay

188 An 82-year-old widow with a clear mind was registered blind and took up temporary accommodation in a residential home.

What was the best way to help her early days in the home?
A contact Guide Dogs for the Blind
B ask an occupational therapist to visit her to help in orientation and accident avoidance
C organise Braille lessons
D ensure that the woman is registered blind so that she could make benefit claims
E supply a mobile phone

189 After 60 years of professional golf, Henry Cotton became too infirm to play. He became insomniac and depressed – Geriatric Depression Scale (GDS) 7/15 (moderately depressed). He was treated with citalopram 10 mg daily for 6 weeks, leading to a GDS of 11/15 (severe depression). The citalopram dose was doubled and a month later the GDS was 10/15.

What was a suitable next stage?
A ask for cognitive behavioural therapy – waiting time is 7 months
B double citalopram
C change to fluoxetine
D refer for ECT
E change to a serotonin/noradrenaline reuptake inhibitor (SNRI)

190 Ms Quick Trip, who was a child in the 1930s, fell a few times over a month. She usually used a stick. There were no neurological signs.

Which of the following investigations were not, at least at first, required?
A x-ray cervical spine and brain
B lying and standing blood pressure measurements
C thyroid function tests
D check footwear
E ask where she kept falling

191 An 80-year-old woman presented with an 18-month history of intermittent, gradually worsening, dysphagia. This was more troublesome with solid foods. Eating took longer; she had lost 3 kg over the previous year. She continued to take ranitidine for control of reflux symptoms.

What was the most likely explanation?
A pharyngeal carcinoma
B pharyngeal pouch
C oesophageal carcinoma
D scleroderma
E achalasia

192 Miss Joan Hunter Dunn had severe Parkinson's disease and had been admitted with aspiration pneumonia. Before transfer to a care home, the ward sister questioned whether advanced care planning would be appropriate.

What would be the best setting in which such a discussion could be held?
A when she is next admitted to her local Care of the Elderly (CoE) unit
B as soon as her admission to the care home, in the hope of avoiding any further hospital admission with aspiration of feeds
C in the GP's surgery
D in the care home, with the help of her case manager, community matron and GP
E in an outpatient clinic with the registrar's help

193 Which of the following is one of the big 'I's' of the non-specific patterns of presentation of illness in the elderly?
A incapacity
B instability
C indecisive
D involutional
E inflexible

194 Which of the following is less than ideal concerning the feeding of an adult who, for safety in swallowing, requires fluids thickened to custard consistency?
A using a tablespoon
B several small meals rather than 2 or 3 large meals per day
C relaxing background classical music playing
D limited conversation between feeder and person being fed
E position of the individual at 45° with the head and neck upright and the chin tucked in

195 Mr Bull, aged 80 years, developed tense blisters on his limbs, trunk and flexures. They tended to develop on normal healthy skin and passed into a chronic intermittent phase which lasted 4 years. Prednisolone 10–25 mg was required to suppress the condition. The blisters, if not infected, healed without leaving scars.

What was Mr Bull's diagnosis?
A bullous pemphigoid
B pemphigus vulgaris
C dermatitis herpetiformis
D erythema multiforme/linear IgA disorder
E pompholyx

196 When setting up a Liverpool Care Pathway (LCP), the ward doctor should:

A discuss the Pathway with a relative or carer

B stop any unrequired previously prescribed medicines

C appreciate that the LCP may be set aside if the patient's health rallies

D bear in mind that a dry mouth may well be a consequence of the drugs in E

E prescribe midazolam, diamorphine and cyclizine to be infused subcutaneously using three different syringes

197 A 76-year-old-man became increasingly breathless.

Chest examination:

1 left hemithorax movements reduced

2 percussion note dull

3 breath sounds reduced over lower half of lung

4 tactile vocal fremitus reduced over lower half of lung

These features suggested?

A left lower lobe consolidation

B left pneumothorax

C left effusion

D bronchopneumonia

E left lower lobe bronchiectasis

198 Which one of the following is not a standard indication for digoxin?

A a sedentary person aged 79 with atrial fibrillation

B an active person aged 79 with atrial fibrillation

C a person aged 79 with a TSH of 0.5 and atrial fibrillation

D heart failure with an ischaemic cardiomyopathy with atrial fibrillation

E an inactive person aged 79 with diastolic heart failure with atrial fibrillation

199 Which one of the following is a contraindication to percutaneous endoscopic gastrostomy in a man of 78 years?

A chiefly lower motor neuron (LMN) signs in a patient with bulbar involvement

B chiefly upper motor neuron (UMN) signs in a patient with bulbar involvement

C three or more aspiration pneumonias

D MMSE of 15–20/30

E vital capacity about 35% of predicted when free of lung infection for 6 weeks

200 In the older person, which of the following is not a potential indicator of underlying malignancy?

A dermatomyositis

B Muehrke's striae

C generalised puritis

D acanthosis nigricans

E acquired ichthyosis

201 A 79-year-old woman consulted her GP because of 8 days of painless swelling over her long-inserted pacemaker generator. The skin was indurated below the generator but not red.

What was the correct course of action?

A get a chest x-ray

B reassure the woman

C request an ultrasound study

D take blood for culture

E prescribe flucloxacillin 1 g qds for a week

202 An 88-year-old Asian man with Alzheimer's (language adjusted MMSE 14/30) began dragging his right foot and two weeks later the left foot. His wife thought that his upper back had 'bent forward' and that there was a 'lump' at the site of angulation. He had developed urinary incontinence.

Examination: a mid-thoracic gibbous; spastic paraparesis; hyperreflexia in legs with extensor plantars; sensory loss below D6.

MRI: complete loss of vertebral bodies D5/6. Intervertebral disc preserved with fluid replacing vertebral bodies.

What was the diagnosis?

A metastatic cancer

B osteoporotic collapse

C tuberculous infection

D myeloma deposits

E *Staphylococcus aureus* infection

203 Concerning 'fuel-poor households'; which of the following apply?

A part of the 'old, cold and elderly' social stigma

B there is an automatic age-related fuel supplement

C the all-cause death rate of people > 80 years old

D concerns the occupants of those households who have to spend more than 10% of their income on heating

E is related to the winter increase in community-acquired pneumonia incidence and prevalence in the elderly population

204 An elderly husband brought his even more elderly wife to a geriatric clinic. The wife had an atrophic glossitis, was agitated, distractible and had a symmetrical peripheral neuropathy.

Blood tests: pancytopenia and mild hyperbilirubinaemia.

What was the clinic working diagnosis?
A aplastic anaemia
B vitamin B_{12} lack
C cerebral atrophy
D myelofibrosis
E acute leukaemia

205 Seventy-seven-year-old George Goget enjoyed a long weekend in Amsterdam. The day he returned he developed stinging dysuria with quantities of yellowish penile discharge.

What was the most likely diagnosis?
A non-specific urethritis
B gonorrhoea
C urinary tract infection
D chlamydia
E herpes simplex infection

206 At the age of 80, Charles Sugar had little interest in controlling his type 2 diabetes.

Drugs: amlodipine, ramipril, aspirin, a statin and maximum doses of metformin and gliclazide – all taken erratically.

Examination: BP 150/94; vision 6/6 bilaterally; neovascularisation of both optic discs.

Investigations:

HbA_{1c}	64 (8.0%)
creatinine	170
Urine albumin:creatinine ratio:	65

What was the first step in management?
A add a daily basal dose of insulin glargine
B add twice-daily insulin detemir
C prescribe doxazosin
D ask for a renal physician's help
E request an ophthalmological review

207 Dr Ready, the GP of 83-year-old Rose Flower, was called to visit by neighbours who had noted noisy behaviour for 2 days. Rose would not let Dr Ready into her home, so a social worker had to be called who used the authority of the Mental Health Act 2007 to gain admission.

Which section of the Act allows such action?
A 11
B 7
C 5
D 3
E 1

208 Regarding age-related changes of the upper gut – which of the following is incorrect?
A the mouth to stomach time for a food bolus is increased
B the P450 enzymes have slowed functions
C hypochlorhydria is infrequent
D gastric H^+ secretion rates are maintained
E gastric emptying time falls with ageing

209 Which of the following may be used by an Occupational Therapist in deciding what modifications, if any, are required in a woman's assessment before she returns from hospital to her home?
A Gleason Score
B Waterlow Score
C Bristol number
D Barthel index
E Fried criteria

210 In his mid-70s, Peter Adams had to be admitted to a nursing home because his long-standing Parkinson's disease made it impossible for him to continue to live alone. He had become forgetful, dysphagic and aggressive. At night he wandered, tended to fall and his aggression worsened. Haloperidol was helpful for staff and fellow patients. Six months later it was noted that he made chewing, pouting and lip-smacking movements and at times there were choreiform movements.

What was Peter Adam's diagnosis?
A tardive dyskinesia
B disorientation in the nursing home
C multiple small vessel strokes
D natural progression of his disease
E Lewy Body disease

211 At annual review a practice Sister found that a 74-year-old man had a BP of 160/105. She asked the GP to see him. At the consultation the next day: BP 175/110.

Investigations: normal urine and ECG; BM 6.5

What was the correct managerial step?
A organise a 24-hour ambulatory BP profile – waiting time 17 to 23 days
B get a repeat reading by the Sister in a week
C prescribe bendroflumethiazide 2.5 mg daily
D prescribe amlodipine 5 mg daily
E refer to the local general medical outpatient clinic

212 Select an error regarding the edentulous state
A is social class related
B is becoming less frequent
C may impair the quality of life
D can impair oral hygiene
E is to be preferred in the very old

213 Gwen Law, a frail 82-year-old (MMSE 15/30) much wanted to return to her home from hospital. Her Barthel index: 10/20. Her sole carers – infirm husband and granddaughter – wanted her home. They declined any additional state-funded help and refused the MDT's offer to provide a commode, hospital bed and hoist. There was an impasse because MDT staff were unwilling for Mrs Law to go to an inadequately prepared and staffed home.

How were matters progressed and what were the options?
A allow Mrs Law to be taken home without additional help
B contact risk assessment staff
C arrange a best interests meeting
D organise discharge to the MDT's choice of nursing home
E take advice from the hospital solicitor

214 Sir Peregrine Charles Tyrwhitt fukes-Humphrey KCMG remained a stickler for correct dress (three-piece pinstripe suit, stiff collar, old Etonian tie, lapel carnation, highly polished black Oxford brogues) even 20 years after retiring from a senior post in the Cabinet Office. Latterly he had had a few 'faints' when looking up to club servants whilst ordering post-prandial port.

What was the diagnosis?
A benign positional vertigo
B recurrent Stokes-Adams attacks
C sick sinus syndrome
D carotid sinus syndrome
E hind brain vascular insufficiency

215 The very elderly (about 85; no accurate record) Puspa Patel left her remote Indian village ostensibly for a few months' visit to her extended family in Leicester, but she knew that she would never return. Her health faltered with loss of weight and frequency of micturition.

Investigations were non-contributory save for: normochromic, normocytic anaemia; CRP 45–60 and a sterile pyuria.

What was the most likely diagnosis?
A transitional cell carcinoma of bladder
B papillary necrosis
C tuberculosis
D myeloma
E schistosomiasis

216 Which of the following pairs are not orthoses?
A shoe raises and depth shoes
B cervical collars and corsets
C knee splints and ankle boots
D dentures and cosmetic nose replacements
E lumbar belts and groin trusses

217 William Withering developed heart failure in his late seventies and subsequently saw yellow/green rings around lights in his home.

Which of the following medications may be responsible?
A captopril
B eplerenone
C digoxin
D bisoprolol
E furosemide with amiloride

218 Around her 74th birthday Miss Iris Spy found that traffic road signs became more difficult to read. This matter was most prominent in crepuscular lighting conditions. In her 75th year, because of progressive visual acuity decline she consulted an ophthalmic surgeon who made a diagnosis and recommended treatment. The diagnosis was?

A chronic simple (primary open-angle) glaucoma

B type II diabetes

C cataracts

D retinitis pigmentosa

E age-related macular degeneration

219 Jimmy McDonald had worked in a Clyde dockyard building marine boiler rooms for 50 years. At the age of 82 years his dyspnoea (COPD: 50 pack year cigarettes) worsened considerably.

Examination: clubbed; large left pleural effusion; sats 85% on air.

What was the likely diagnosis?

A left heart failure

B lung cancer

C post-pneumonic effusion

D mesothelioma

E cor pulmonale

220 Concerning the feet of elderly people, which one of the following is not applicable?

A onchocerciasis

B onycholysis

C onychogryphosis

D onychomycosis

E onychocryptosis

221 Which of the following features is suggestive of frailty according to the Fried criteria?

A dyspnoea

B loss of height

C slow movements

D depression

E dementia

222 Which of the 5 following choices best describes the widespread use of a β-lactam and macrolide combination for treatment of community-acquired pneumonias?
A the combination allows reduction in the frequency of administration
B the combination allows reduction in dose of the individual antibiotics
C the combination increases the spectrum of activity
D the combination therapy reduces the total length of treatment
E together they are synergistic against the common pneumonic pathogens

223 Mr Yassim Ali (born 1356 thus according to the muslim calender, making him 77 years old in 2012) was a devout Muslim. He took the following drugs: aspirin, a statin, a β-blocker, insulin, a long-acting nitrate and an ACEI. He asked his doctor for advice regarding a visit to Mecca – it is compulsory, finances permitting, for every Muslim to undertake this pilgrimage once in a lifetime.

Examination: proliferative retinopathy; no pulses below femorals.

Investigations: HbA_{1c} 7.5 (59)
                  eGFR   35

What was the most suitable comment regarding the planned trip?
A go and take a helper with you
B infirmity may be used to exempt a potential Mecca pilgrim
C visit during the Saudi cool months
D take an umbrella
E act on WHO vaccination recommendations before departure

224 At which of the following regions do osteoporotic vertebral fractures most commonly occur?
A mid to lower cervical
B upper thoracic
C thoracolumbar
D midlumbar
E lumbosacral

225 June Woodland, aged 74, was known to have aortic and mitral valve regurgitation and was sent up to a clinic because of 3 weeks of tiredness and failure to thrive. Her GP had found her bilirubin to be 42 and her eGFR had fallen from 48 to 34 over 8 weeks.

What was the likely diagnosis?
A heart failure
B subacute bacterial endocarditis
C cholecystitis
D hepatitis
E urinary infection

226 Thomas Crapper (born 1935) had been 'a martyr to my stomach' for many years. He had been diagnosed as having 'irritable bowel' but when he developed weight loss and diarrhoea and was found to be iron deficient he was 'topped and tailed'. Multiple biopsies were taken from normal-looking mucosa in stomach, duodenum and colon. The finding of stunted, atrophic villi led to a request for a specific blood test.

What was the diagnosis?
A gastro-oesophageal reflux disease
B microscopic colitis
C inflammatory bowel disease
D chronic pancreatitis
E coeliac disease

227 Mr Black's watch malfunctioned. It continued to stop despite being declared mechanically intact by the manufacturers. He realised that his watch arm had stopped swinging when he walked. He had physical signs suggesting dysfunction of the substantia nigra. Which drug allowed satisfactory restitution of his automatic winding facility?
A d-penicillamine
B propranolol
C polyethylene glycol
D levodopa
E risperidone

228 In Dolcimedland, situated on the north Mediterranean coast, there was a high proportion of old people. Which of the following best explained the ageing of the Dolcimedlander population?
A sound preventive medical care systems
B people live longer – 'good DNA'
C their Mediterranean diet
D first class hospitals
E families having fewer children

229 Mrs Sphere, a golf- and bowls-playing 74-year-old, took twice-daily 30/70 mixed insulin. There were some isolated hypoglycaemic episodes.

Her average home blood sugar figures:	pre-breakfast	13.5
	pre-lunch	3.5
	pre-supper	11.7
	bedtime	6.7

Which of the following strategies was the most appropriate?
A   reduce her morning biphasic isophane insulin
B   increase her morning biphasic isophane insulin
C   change to insulin detemir twice daily
D   add a few units of insulin aspart at bedtime
E   change to a basal bolus insulin regime of glargine and lispro insulins

230 Regarding the Attendance Allowance, which of the following is correct?
A   only claimable for those aged 65 years and more
B   is means tested
C   may be claimed if claimant is in hospital
D   is a short-term benefit
E   applies to 'office hours' help only

231 Because of head banging, repetitive purposeless behaviour, grunting and wandering, 68-year-old Ronald Brewer (RB) earned a long-term elderly mentally infirm (EMI) placement. His son-in-law and daughter had to inspect and pass the planned home before RB was transferred. Before inspection they took a 3-week holiday in Cadiz. Towards the end of that period a message came that they were prolonging their stay. At some stage they returned to England, never visited their relative and did not respond to repeated hospital efforts to contact them. RB was blocking a bed in a care of the elderly rehabilitation ward.

What had to be done?
A   accept the status quo, perhaps for some years
B   aim to place RB in an establishment with a warden and day and night package of care
C   ask the police to locate the relatives
D   try for an admission to a long-stay psychiatric unit
E   activate the hospital legal system for authority to effect an EMI unit transfer

232 A man of 80 years suddenly found that he could not walk.

Examination showed 5/5 power in the arms and 0/5 in his legs. There was a sensory level at the umbilicus.

At what level was the lesion?
A C4
B T4
C D10
D L1
E L3

233 A 75-year-old woman developed a fixed, clearly defined red crusting rash involving her perineal and vulval areas. She was otherwise well, took no regular medicines and enjoyed cooking for her men friends. Over 6 months her rash extended by a few millimetres, but failed to respond to emollients, potent topical steroids and antifungal creams.

Which was the likely diagnosis?
A vulval eczema
B squamous cell carcinoma
C extramammary Paget's disease
D acrodermatitis enteropathica
E cutaneous candidiasis

234 The belly pain/discomfort of a 73-year-old man with a diagnosis of pancreatic carcinoma with liver and omental deposits no longer responded to paracetamol (acetaminophen).

What was the next step in analgesia?
A PRN oral morphine
B codeine phosphate
C paracetamol and codeine
D gabapentin and codeine
E fentanyl patches

235 Faecal leaking developed in a man of 75 who, for the past few years had successfully taken an unchanged dose of tablets containing levodopa + carbidopa.

What was the most likely explanation?
A constipation with overflow
B parkinsonism autonomic neuropathy
C Parkinson's plus syndrome
D colorectal carcinoma
E side-effect of co-careldopa

236 Pyrophosphate arthropathy:
  A usually affects knee joints
  B may be precipitated by trauma or severe medical illness
  C may mimic septic arthritis
  D intra-articular dexamethasone is of use
  E joint x-rays are unhelpful in an established case

237 Which of the following suggest that a patient's competency (capacity) should be assessed?
  A 90+ years
  B a nursing home resident of 5 years standing
  C a dishevelled appearance
  D infection-related delirium
  E none of the above

238 What is a suitable clinical approach to non-diabetic men of 80–85 years with sustained blood pressures of ≥ 150/100 without target organ damage?
  A treat all of them and hope to extend their lives
  B treat none of them and avoid drug damage
  C treat some
  D check for secondary causes of hypertension
  E ask a friend

239 A 76-year-old woman is 'tired'. Physical examination is normal. BP 138/88; PFR: 350 L/min.

Investigations:

Hb	11.8
MCV	90
CRP	3
TSH	7.5
FT4	14.9 (10 – 25)

What was the correct course?
  A supply thyroxine
  B prescribe carbimazole
  C request a further TSH assay in 3 months
  D advise 3 months of iron tablets
  E do nothing

240 What is the principal cause of retinal blindness in the UK?
A age-related macular degeneration
B retinitis pigmentosa
C cataracts
D glaucoma
E diabetes

241 As per NICE's (2011) recommendations, perindopril 8 mg/day was prescribed because a 76-year-old patient's BP was 148/109. After a week the BP was 128/92 but the eGFR had halved and plasma K^+ was 0.9 mmol/L above the reference range.

What was the likely explanation?
A over-rapid BP control leading to renal hypoperfusion
B unilateral renal infarction
C developing renal failure
D renal artery stenosis: fibromuscular dysplasia type
E renal artery stenosis: arteriosclerotic type

242 An 85-year-old woman was seen in an ED because of increased confusion and 3 falls over the previous 8 days.

Drugs: aspirin, simvastatin, gutt timolol, gliclazide, bendroflumethiazide, omeprazole.

Examination: slow SR; PB 165/85; no other abnormal findings.

Investigations: plasma electrolytes within reference ranges; Hb 10.7; MCV 85; urine dip: nitrite positive. Rhythm strip: complete heart block.

What was the probable explanation of the confusion and falls?
A heart failure
B drug side-effect
C urine infection
D renal failure
E anaemia

243 A multi-centred pan-European trial was performed to investigate the effects of a monoclonal antibody in patients with resected colorectal cancer but with distant metastases. Half of the 5000 patients received 8 months of monoclonal infusions and the remaining 2500 best supportive therapy. The principal outcome was cancer-related death. The median survival time was 9.5 months in the supportive therapy and 11.5 months in the biological therapy patients. These periods correspond to a Kaplan-Meier probability of 0.5.

Which of the following best describes the survival time of the intervention group patients?
A immune therapy was applied for 11 months and 15 days
B 0.5 is the probability of surviving 11½ months or more if treated with the monoclonal antibody
C 50% of the intervention group were alive 11½ months after starting treatment
D the economy of the best supportive care group medicine implies that such treatment is sensible
E the cost of monoclonal therapy is justified by the enhanced survival

244 Which of the following x-ray reports phrases suggested an urgent referral to a thoracic unit?
A Honda sign
B lesion in the widow area
C cobblestone appearance
D coin lesion
E string sign

245 Charles Dreadnought consulted because of not feeling well for the last 6 months despite taking an escalating list of 'over the counter' superstore 'health enhancing remedies' which included zinc, selenium and magnesium supplements, vitamin C, strong vitamin B compound tablets, St John's wort, folic acid, cod liver oil, garlic and glucosamine.

Physical examination did not further matters. Blood tests: Hb, liver, thyroid, electrolyte, renal and CRP values within reference ranges for a 79-year-old chap.

What was a sensible approach to this man's circumstances?
A prescribe citalopram
B suggest stopping the superstore pills
C prescribe iron and vitamin C capsules
D access cogitative behavioural therapy
E wish him well – 'the blood tests are OK'

246 The extended role of the occupational therapist includes which of the following?
  A assessment of cognitive function post-brain attack
  B contributing to rehabilitation goal setting and discharge planning
  C has access to funds to pay patient's TV and dog licences
  D use Waterlow and Gleeson scores from the Blue Book
  E help choose respite care in residential and nursing homes

247 The long-retired Jean Collie had to be admitted with community-acquired pneumonia.

Observations: temperature 38.5° C; pulse 115; respirations 34; BP 85/58 mm Hg.

Investigations: wbc   18 with 92% pmns
                 urea   8.7

What was her CURB-65 score?
  A 5
  B 4
  C 3
  D 2
  E 1

248 An 80-year-old woman was brought in by ambulance with palpitations, dyspnoea at rest and borderline syncope. Her heart was in a regular rhythm at 150 bpm. The ECG showed a broad-complex monomorphic tachycardia with a QRS duration of 150 ms (100).

Which of the following is the most likely to support a diagnosis of a ventricular tachycardia?
  A diastolic BP 85–90
  B ventricular rate ≥ 200
  C past history of myocardial infarction
  D hypokalaemia
  E Brugada syndrome

249 A 77-year-old man's urine darkened and his GP referred him to a geriatric same day assessment unit because of the following results:

bilirubin	44
AST	120
ALT	85
AP	70

Which of the following drugs was most likely to have induced the hepato-cellular damage?
A amiodarone
B amlodipine
C aspirin
D atenolol
E atorvastatin

250 Which of the following is a diagnosis?
A constipation
B failure to cope
C found on floor
D recurrent falls
E BIBA

251 A man of 87, who lived alone, had early Alzheimer's; MMSE 22/30. He tended to leave the gas cooker burning when he was out of the house. He strongly denied that this was dangerous and wished to leave the ward, having recovered from a urinary infection.

What was the correct course for the ward staff to take?
A because his MMSE was 22 he did not have mental capacity and had to be kept safely away from his home
B a social worker had to decide where to place him.
C a best interests meeting had to be convened
D he had capacity and could do as he wished
E he had to sign himself out of the hospital against medical advice

252 Aged 72, John Smith developed a lobar pneumonia with rusty sputum. Treatment that evening began with standard community-acquired pneumonia antibiotics. The following morning sputum microscopy showed Gram-positive diplococcic and similar organisms were grown from sputum and both blood culture bottles.

To which appropriate antibiotic was John Smith changed?
A benzylpenicillin
B flucloxacillin
C gentamycin
D metronidazole
E clindamycin

253 Mr Cliff Edge, aged 82, was sent urgently to a 'hot case' geriatric clinic because he had become unwell over the previous 6 weeks, with loss of energy, weight and appetite for no obvious reason.

Past history: ischaemic heart disease. Drugs: digoxin 250, furosemide 40, warfarin, simvastatin 40.

Examination: wt 51 kg; BMI 23; AF: BP 84/55; no signs of failure.

What was the correct clinical decision?
A stop all drugs
B stop all drugs except for warfarin
C substitute digoxin with atenolol
D arrange admission to hospital
E phone a friend

254 Which of the following is or are incorrect regarding an OGGT?
A defined in terms of a 75g oral glucose load
B the diagnosis of diabetes is secure if 2 hour plasma glucose concentration is ≥ 11.1
C is needed if HbA_{1c} is 9. 5 (80)
D is needed if fasting glucose in older people lies between ≥ 6.1 and ≤ 6.9
E identifies those people with impaired glucose tolerance (plasma glucose at 2 hours between ≥ 7.8 and < 11.1)

255 Elderly septic patients are frequently dehydrated and oliguric. Which one of the following suggests a pre-renal (physiological) oliguria was present in contrast to intrinsic renal failure (ARF/AKI)?
A microscopic erythrocytes
B red cell casts
C plasma osmolality of 280 mOsm/L
D urine Na^+ > 20 mmol/L
E urine Na^+ < 20 mmol/L

256 Deafness is classified as conductive or sensory (or mixed). The differentiation is made by using tuning fork tests – Rene's and Weber's. In testing the hearing, which of the following is correct?

A Rinne's test is positive if AC > BC

B Rinne's test is positive if BC > AC

C Rinne's procedure tests cochlea function

D Rinne's procedure tests sensorineural function

E Weber's test detects cochlear and auditory dysfunction

257 Which of the following liver images are compatible with the following fasting blood figures?

triglycerides	5.4
ALT	175
HbA$_{1c}$	9 (75)
ACR	95

A biliary stones

B cirrhosis

C normal findings

D fatty infiltration

E prominent lobar septae

258 Bruce Quercus boxed for the British Army during his National Service (1952–54) and then fought professionally for 12 years. At 80, Mrs Quercus realised that her husband had slowed down and walked with a shuffle.

Medical history: atrial fibrillation; ischaemic heart disease, hypertension; T2DM.

Examination: increased tone in legs but not in arms. Bradykinesia. The 'Get Up and Go' test took more than 35 seconds. The gait was wide based.

What was the likely diagnosis?

A Lewy Body disease

B chronic subdural bleeds

C idiopathic PD

D vascular Parkinson's

E dementia pugilistica

259 Consider a man of 80 years who for 8 months was thought to be depressed (GDS 8/15) and had AD (MMSE 17/30).

What was the best therapeutic choice?
A sertraline
B midodrine
C no tablets
D citalopram
E fluoxetine

260 Why is the average dose of warfarin needed to keep an INR at a set value less for a person aged 75 than 25 years?
A smaller liver mass with increasing age
B smaller volume of distribution
C increased first pass metabolism
D reduced glomerular filtration rate (GFR) with increasing age
E reduced numbers of binding sites

261 An 83-year-old man was admitted with palpitations and New York Class III dyspnoea (dyspnoea of minimal effort).

chest x-ray: generalised cardiomegaly; cardiothoracic ratio 70%; upper lobe diversion; Kerley B lines and bilateral effusions.

left ventricular ejection fraction: 20%
B natriuretic peptide: 8500

What was the likely cardiac diagnosis?
A dilated cardiomyopathy
B Chagas' disease
C cardiac amyloid
D ischaemic cardiomyopathy
E right ventricular cardiomyopathy

262 In his late 70s, George Grumble developed 'indigestion' which took him to his GP. He was prescribed omeprazole but, because of no improvement, returned to the surgery after 20 days. Which of the following is not regarded as an alarm (red flag) feature?
A no response to the PPI
B weight loss
C dysphagia
D iron deficiency
E previous gastric ulcer

263 Identify a risk factor which carries the least increased chance of prolonged grieving after the death of a relative.
A close kinship with the deceased
B loss of income
C death of a spouse
D suicide of a family member
E unexpected death

264 The majority of dementing brains lose volume. Which of the following would be the most appropriate radiological technique to assess differential brain volume changes in an 84-year-old man who could recall items after a delay but scored less well in orientation, naming and calculation? MMSE: 25/30.

Standard dementia screen blood variables and a CXR showed no abnormalities.
A structural CT brain imaging with contrast
B ^{18}FDG-PET scan
C T2-weighted MRI sequences
D T1-weighted MRI sequences
E FLAIR weighted MRI sequences

265 Mrs Tar noticed that her husband Jack, who after naval service had worked in the dockyard to the age of 50 years – was 'different'. His memory was reliable but he had non-threatening hallucinations concerning unknown people who daily visited him at home, stayed until 5 p.m., then left leaving no trace of their visit. A CT brain showed prominent global brain loss. Medicines: none.

What was the diagnosis?
A Alzheimer's dementia (AD)
B fronto-temporal dementia (FTD)
C Lewy Body dementia (LBD)
D semantic dementia (SD)
E vascular dementia (VD)

266 The end-stage consequences of long-term nicotine addiction – dyspnoea, pain, fatigue and low mood are very common in people with COPD and lung cancer.

Which of the following should contribute least to a 'good death'?
A MDT holistic help with patients' needs
B palliative care staff
C morphia and benzodiazepines
D ferrous sulphate and folate for concomitant anaemia
E PRN oxygen

267 Edmundo Mos had recurrent attacks of joint pains such that he could not conduct his BBC band. Each attack involved pain and swelling of one or two joints. The attacks were sudden and lasted 12–24 hours, occurring every 4–6 weeks. Different joints were involved in separate attacks.

What was the most likely diagnosis?
A calcium pyrophosphate arthropathy
B gout
C osteoarthritis
D palindromic rheumatism
E rheumatoid arthritis

268 Mye Badluck was unfortunate that despite an INR in the region of 2.2–2.8 for the previous 5 months, a clot formed in his left atrium. CT imaging showed that a clot had impacted, causing ischaemic obstruction to the distal quarter of the middle cerebral artery. At 68 minutes after the brain attack a decision had to be made regarding the use of recombinant tissue plasminogen activator (rt-PA). INR 2.5.

Which of the following was the correct next step?
A infuse a full dose of rt-PA over 60 minutes
B use a half dose of rt-PA
C rt-PA contraindicated
D infuse unfractionated heparin
E best supportive care

269 Dr Charles Pooter's last telephone words to Miss B Quick were 'Bea, take three each day and have your blood checked on New Year's Eve. Happy Christmas. Ciao'. Bea Quick bled to death on 28/12/2012.

What had gone wrong?
A high-dose cooking sherry is a comfort at times of isolation in cold weather
B she received and took amoxicillin from her local A & E for 'bronchitis' which started on 24/12/2012
C she confused a 3 mg dose of warfarin with 3 × 5 mg tablets and took the latter
D her arthritis 'played up' but over the counter analgesics (aspirin and ibuprofen compound tablets) fixed it with regular doses
E repeated applications of vodka and cranberry juice helped the lonely days of the Festive Season to pass

270 Mr Hardy Mater, in his 80s, was no more than a little forgetful. He had been anticoagulated for 5 years on account of a mitral valve prolapse complicated by atrial fibrillation. Drugs: digoxin, simvastatin, furosemide and warfarin. He slipped and hit his head on a shelf in a superstore.

The admitting SHO recorded grasping respiration, a GCS of 4 (E1, V1, M2) and fixed dilated pupils.

What was the MAU SHO's working diagnosis?
A subarachnoid bleed
B subdural bleed
C pontine bleed
D frontal lobe bleed
E meningeal artery bleed

271 In the context of the last weeks of life, which of the following is correct?
A generally for the terminally ill, fear of a painful death ranks before fear of dying
B those members of the palliative care team with strong religious beliefs should talk about their faith to their dying patients and offer to pray with them
C It is always better to die in hospital than in one's home
D a palliative care unit is fertile ground for a religious proselytiser
E spirituality is defined in terms of the core beliefs of the person under discussion

272 An asymptomatic 80-year-old woman attended a 'well woman' clinic at which her dipstick urine was positive for leukocyte esterase but negative for nitrites. Which of the following apply?
A the observation has no prognostic value
B there are similar findings in 20–30% of 80-year-old women
C the benefit of treatment outweighs any consequence
D treatment should eradicate any bacteria
E matters are different in older men

273 Sid Weal, an ex-HGV driver, had a brain attack which left him sharp of ear and eye but slow of mind. He asked his GP whether he should continue to drive his Ford. Which of the following are pertinent?
A advise that he surrender his driving licence
B advise to drive only in good daylight
C seek advice from the UK Driver and Vehicle Licensing Authority
D mention that all drivers are very likely to have accidents by the age of 83
E tell him that occasional taxis are cheaper than maintaining a car

274 Mrs Jones, an outgoing, spry 75-year-old woman, was found in her home shuddering, distraught and moaning. From disturbance to her clothing it appeared that she had been sexually molested.

What had to be set going?
A genital examination in her bedroom
B take genital swabs
C take her for a shower
D ring social services while she was being taken to the local ED
E arrange for urgent post-exposure HIV prophylaxis

275 Robert Platt attended his GP's surgery for a medical following his 75th birthday. He was well and only took an occasional paracetamol (acetaminophen). The practise Sister and the GP later found his BP to be in the region of 170/90.

What was the best decision regarding the BP?
A do nothing – the BP will settle
B re-measure the BP in a few weeks
C request a 24-hour ambulatory BP monitor
D prescribe a CCB
E prescribe an ACEI

276 A to E list pairs of features which, except for one pair, historically help separate a vasovagal event from cardiac syncope. Which one is the rogue pair?

Event	Vaso-vagal	Cardiac
A older age	less common	more common
B onset	gradual	sudden
C nausea	common	unlikely
D fatigue	occurs	rare
E incontinence	uncommon	uncommon

277 In an elderly person with a Pancoast's tumour, which of the following may not be found?
A croaky voice
B partial ptosis
C exophthalmos
D meiosis
E ipsilateral anhydrosis

278 An 83-year-old man with agitated depression developed a dry mouth and restless leg movements. Which of the following was most likely to have caused the dyskinesia?

A atenolol

B carbamazepine

C citalopram

D haloperidol

E quetiapine

279 While a 77-year-old man with an acute hemiparesis and atrial fibrillation was being admitted, a fire broke out in the CT scanning suite. The service had to be halted for an unknown number of hours.

What was the best course of action?

A subcutaneous low molecular weight heparin

B wait for the CT service to resume

C arrange for urgent transfer to a neighbouring facility

D give aspirin

E give aspirin with dipyridamole

280 Regarding visual acuity in the elderly; which of the following is incorrect?

A 20/20 vision and 6/6 vision mean something different

B the numerator in the visual acuity equation is a distance approximating to infinity

C the denominator in the visual acuity equation is the distance at which the test letters or symbols can be seen with 'normal' or corrected vision

D impairment of visual acuity is multifactorial, involving changes in one or more of cornea, lens, vitreal fluid or macula

E presbyopia is always pathological

281 Steven Coe, aged 78 years, was referred from an orthopaedic clinic to a metabolic physician 'because the knee and tibial discomfort are not surgical conditions'.

Investigations: Fbc, eGFR, electrolytes and CRP: normal; isoenzyme analysis of a much raised alkaline phosphate showed that it predominantly came from bone. LFTs: normal. Hip and tibial x-rays showed a mixture of lytic and sclerotic changes.

What was the likely diagnosis?

A healing undisplaced fractures

B metastatic cancer

C Paget's disease

D osteosarcoma

E osteomalacia

282 An 88-year-old woman was admitted because she had become 'off her feet'. Her Alzheimer's was advancing, donepezil was no longer of help (MMSE 13/30).

Investigations: creatinine   889
                  K^+ 5.3

What was the correct first step?
A ultrasound of the renal tract
B catheterise for CSU and accurate fluid balance
C await further data and details
D request dialysis
E complete a DNAR form

283 Elderly people have to face their death and the death of family and friends more frequently than others. Which of the following is not a risk factor for an abnormal grief response?
A active or past mental depression
B suddenly becoming an elderly widower
C maintenance of mobility and external interests
D having cared for the deceased during the final illness for 6+ months
E low self-esteem and social support

284 The report of an unenhanced brain MRI performed on an 80-year-old man contained the following: 'dilated ventricles, cortical atrophy, enlarged sulci, medial temporal lobe atrophy, prominent hippocampal atrophy, calcification of falx cerebri'.

What was the probable conclusion of the report?
A normal pressure hydrocephalus
B fronto-temporal dementia
C Alzheimer's dementia
D limbic encephalitis
E ischaemic cerebrovascular disease

285 The asymptomatic and active Mrs Strongbone was diagnosed as having primary hyperparathyroidism (Ca^{2+} 2.9; PTH × 4 above reference range; eGFR 55). Fifteen months later, on her 86th birthday, she was found to have a serum Ca^{2+} of 3.0.

What was the correct step to take?
A prescribe a bisphosphonate
B prescribe a bisphosphonate with cinacalcet
C arrange for a bone densitometry measurement
D arrange for parathyroid imaging
E refer to an endocrine surgeon

286 In the MRCP PACES examination one of the patients was a 74-year-old woman with extensive psoriasis and abnormal toe nails. Dr Stride was asked to state her diagnosis and then other conditions which might have been related to the nail diagnosis – her diagnosis was?
A clubbing
B koilonychia
C paronychia
D onycholysis
E onychogryphosis

287 The son of a patient with dementia (MMSE 18/30) asked her mother's GP to act as signatory to ratify an advanced care plan (ACP) drafted by his father. The ACP involved granting the son Lasting Power of Attorney.

What was the most appropriate response by the GP?
A agree to sign, provided that a partner of the practice agrees that the ACP content is acceptable
B asses the patient's capacity before a decision
C sign the ACP because it is in the patient's best interests
D suggest that a solicitor be hired
E phone a friend

288 A 79-year-old man had recently received the diagnosis of motor neurone disease on the basis of dysarthria, variable dysphasia, fasciculation in the tongue and a normal brain MRI. Swallowing difficulty increased, at times food particles were expelled via his nostrils. Abbreviated Mental Test (AMT) score 9/10.

What was urgently needed?
A total parenteral nutrition
B percutaneous gastroenterostomy
C draw up end of life plans
D request videofluoroscopy of swallowing
E get speech and language help

289 Concerning tinnitus: which is incorrect?
A often linked with presbycusis
B unrelated to hearing loss
C often idiopathic
D tight relationship with Ménière's disease
E may be related to furosemide treatment

290 Sixty hours after falling from a ladder and sustaining closed fractures of a femoral shaft, tibia and pelvic rami, a 77-year-old man developed a petechial rash on his chest, tachypnea and became disorientated in person and place. He required restraint.

Examination: GCS 12 (E4, V3, M5); no neurological signs.

Investigations:

Hb	9.2
wbc	14
platelets	100
creatinine	147
Na$^+$	130
glucose	9.2
CRP	73
ABG	hypocapnia and hypoxaemia
brain CT	no abnormality
CSF	acellular

What was the likely diagnosis?
A herpes encephalitis
B fat emboli
C limbic encephalitis
D hyponatraemia
E non-convulsive status

291 The left ventricular ejection fraction (LVEF) gives information which helps estimate cardiac prognosis.

Which of the following is correct?
A a normal LVEF is expressed as 100% of heart function
B a result of 50% represents serious dysfunction
C with heart disease, the LVEF inexorably declines
D if the LVEF is normal, heart failure is excluded
E the method of measurement is operator dependent

292 Three weeks into treatment of a nephritis (prednisolone/azathioprine/cyclophosphamide), 75-year-old Mr R Bright developed a sudden very severe headache over the whole of his cranium, passing down to his pectoral girdle.

Examination: GCS 15/15; pulse 116, SR; BP 170/100; normal fundi; bilateral soft, pitting, peripheral oedema; no other signs.

Investigation:

wbc	13.3
CRP	19
platelets	250
albumin	19
CT brain (non-enhanced):	no free blood; hyperdense, cord-like material in the superior sagittal sinus.

What was the diagnosis?
A subarachnoid haemorrhage
B cerebral venous thrombosis
C nephrotic syndrome
D nephritic syndrome
E carotid artery dissection

293 Which of the following tools and techniques should be available in a surgery or A & E department with which to access visual acuity?
A Snellen chart at 6 m or a 3 m reversed Snellen
B Ishihara plates
C finger counting
D hand movements
E torchlight perception

294 The most important advantage of the Chronic Kidney Disease (CKD) staging of renal function facilitates:
A the understanding of measurement of glomerular filtration rate (GFR)
B the timely referral of patients to renal services
C the identification of patients with progressive loss of GFR
D accurate judgment of drug dose at Stages 4 (15–30 ml/minute/m^2 BSA) and 5 (< 15)
E clarifying the non-linearity of serum creatinine concentrations and GFR

295 Under which of the following circumstances may a modified early warning score (MEWS) of 4 not be set aside?
A if the patient is on a Liverpool Care Pathway
B if requested by and documented in the clinical records by the medical staff
C if a competent patient insists on not being disturbed
D if a patient is obviously well, cheerful and eating
E if the MEWS trigger has been reset to 6 for a specific patient

296 An outbreak of diarrhoea and vomiting occurred in a residential home over a 72-hour period. Residents and staff were affected. No source was found; pathogenic bacteria were not recovered from 35 stool samples tested.

Which of the following is the most likely cause of the outbreak?
A *Clostridium difficile*
B *Giardia lamblia*
C staphylococcal food contamination
D enterotoxigenic *Escherichia coli*
E Norovirus

297 Frau Auguste Dietrich was referred to a geriatric outpatient clinic because of increasing memory weakness but was otherwise well. Laboratory dementia screen: no abnormalities. MMSE 22/30 – reduced score due to memory impairment; Addenbrooke's Cambridge Evaluation-revised: 67/100 with loss of memory. Geriatric Depression Score: 2/15 (no depression).

CT brain: age-related involutional changes.

What did the brain MRI show?
A the T2-weighted or fluid-attenuated inversion recovery sequences (FLAIR) showing white matter abnormalities
B hippocampal swelling with hyperintensity
C asymmetrical inferior temporal lobe and hippocampal atrophy
D symmetrical medial temporal lobe volume loss (atrophy) with hippocampal atrophy
E considerable white matter and other ischaemic change with hippocampal atrophy

298 At the age of 38 years, Best Banting developed T1DM. Forty years later he had impaired vision, pain and parenthesis in his legs, erectile dysfunction and began to fall frequently. Drugs: perindopril, simvastatin, indapamide, aspirin, glargine and aspartate insulins.

Examination: BP 140/80 and 100/72 lying and standing, respectively; proliferative retinopathy; sensory loss to knees.

What was the first most appropriate intervention?
A stop indapamide
B do a short Synacthen test
C add midodrine
D order toe to groin elastic stockings
E add fludrocortisone

299 An 86-year-old woman developed idiopathic grand mal epilepsy. Despite using two potent, well-established anti-epileptic drugs prescribed by a specialist neurologist, fits remained too frequent.

Which of the following is the most likely explanation?
A misdiagnosis of epilepsy
B hippocampal sclerosis
C inadequate doses
D poor compliance
E inappropriate choice of drugs

300 Which is the best combination therapy to diminish exacerbations in patients with moderate COPD ($FEV_1 \geq 50\%$ of predicted value) whilst allowing background medications to be taken?
A the antimuscarinic tiotropium 18 µg daily
B the long-acting β_2 agonist salmeterol 50 µg twice daily
C theophylline tablets twice daily dosed to gain a 6-hour trough concentration of 10–20 mg/L
D azithromycin taken for 12 months
E tiotropium 18 µg daily + salmeterol 50 µg twice daily

301 Regarding atrial fibrillation (AF), which is correct?
A assuming no contraindications, all patients with permanent, persistent and paroxysmal AF should be anticoagulated
B the CURB-65 tool helps in risk assessment
C warfarin and aspirin are equally safe
D an INR of 3–4 gives greater protection than lesser degrees of anticoagulation
E about 25% of people >80 years have persistent/permanent AF

302 Wbc 21.5; CRP 189; IgG 0.02 g/L. Given these laboratory findings, what is the best antibiotic treatment of a spreading cellulitis?

A oral clindamycin
B oral flucloxacillin
C oral erythromycin or clarithromycin
D intravenous clindamycin
E intravenous flucloxacillin

303 When he was 80 years old, Tom Forrest, who had been a game keeper for 60 years in Ambridge Park, developed a 'spot' on his right cheek. The 'spot' was well circumscribed, skin coloured and nodular. A few fine blood vessels passed over the lesion – which was?

A a squamous cell carcinoma
B a basal cell carcinoma
C a superficial malignant melanoma
D a nodular melanoma
E an amelanotic melanoma

304 After 5 days of cephalosporin treatment for a presumed urinary tract infection, Mrs Avon Bridge and other members of her nursing home developed *Clostridium difficile* colitis.

Which of the following was unlikely to be true of their stools?

A Bristol type stools 1 to 2 was the main variety passed
B Bristol types 6 and 7 predominated
C daily stool volume was 0.5 to 1.0 L
D stool *C difficile* toxin excretion was prolonged
E stool microscopy showed excessive numbers of white blood cells

305 Which one of the following is not a feature of the autonomic neuropathy of diabetes?

A postural hypotension
B vomiting or diarrhoea or both
C resting tachycardia
D gustatory sweating
E foot ulcers

306 Mrs Thinbones consults because of the results of a BUPA 'Well Elderly' screen her son had arranged for his 75-year-old mother. Abnormalities were a serum total vitamin D 15 nmol/L (> 50) and bone density score of –2.5. The 'Get Up and Go' test took more than 30 seconds.

Which of the following is the likely diagnosis or management?
A hypoparathyroidism
B three months of calcium tablets will suffice
C relax – marginal risk of femoral fracture
D osteoporosis
E osteomalacia

307 Which feature is correct concerning the Attendance Allowance (AA)?
A a medical examination is required
B it cannot be claimed if the client is not receiving external carer help
C the AA is means tested
D it can only be claimed if the client becomes unwell
E it can be claimed even if no one is giving care

308 Ann Sugar, aged 77, visited her GP because of 6 months of weight loss and pruritus vulvae. BMI: 30 kg/m^2.

What was the most likely result of a plasma glucose assay, the blood having been sampled after 14 hours of fasting?
A 3.0
B 5.5
C 6.9
D 9.9
E 17.3

309 A 75-year-old man was knocked off his pushbike and struck his head on a curb. Subsequently he had attacks of vertigo ('like a merry-go-round') followed by being wobbly for the next 10–15 seconds. Symptoms occurred when rolling over in bed, looking upwards or bending down.

Examination: when lying flat there was torsional vertigo to the right, starting at 5 seconds and lasting 10 seconds. This was followed by dizziness.

The diagnosis was?
A binge drinking
B compensation-orientated symptoms
C Ménière's disease
D cochlear dysfunction
E benign paroxysmal positional vertigo

310 A to E show pairs of features which are referable to the historical differentiation of syncope from seizures, save for one, which is?

event	syncope	seizure
A convulsion	common	common
B trigger	common	rare
C onset	gradual	sudden
D tongue biting	rare	common
E recovery	rapid	slow

311 How is the correct length of a supportive walking stick (cane) estimated?
A the distance from the ipsilateral iliac crest to the floor with the subject wearing outdoor shoes
B the distance from the base of the thumb to the floor with the arm held in 15° of abduction
C the distance from the ipsilateral greater trochanter to the floor
D the distance from the contralateral femoral trochanter to the floor, deducting the depth of the ferrule
E the height of the person minus 65% of that height

312 For arthritic pains Mrs Pill took 1g paracetamol (acetaminophen) four times daily (and some over painful nights). She kept her epilepsy controlled with phenytoin 300mg daily. One Christmas Eve she developed influenza for which she took 3 or 4 daily doses of a proprietary compound containing ephedrine hydrochloride, caffeine and paracetamol. On New Year's Day she was taken to hospital jaundiced with extensive petechiae and died.

Blood taken 2 hours before death showed:

bilirubin	75
ALT	1090
PT	80
creatinine	550
lactate	17.9 (0.5 – 2.0)
arterial pH	7.0
paracetamol:	just detected

What was the diagnosis?
A acute influential hepatitis
B portal vein thrombosis
C paracetamol liver failure
D metabolic acidosis
E phenytoin liver failure

313 Various members of all but one of the following groups of drugs have the potential to cause or exacerbate parkinsonism. Which is the odd man out in not having this propensity?
A   dopamine receptor blockers (neuroleptics)
B   atypical antipsychotics
C   phenothiazines
D   monoamine oxidase-B inhibitors
E   substituted benzamides

314 What is the approximate dose in mg, of furosemide, required to produce a dieresis in a normotensive heart failure male aged 80 years who has a eGFR of 12 ml/minute/1.75 m² BSA?
A   40
B   80
C   120
D   180
E   250

315 Mr Ben Ian Gibb, aged 77 years, (BMI 35.5) could not tolerate metformin and failed to get his HbA_{1c} < 7.5 on maximum doses of gliclazide. Blood pressure, heart failure, platelets and cholesterol were well controlled. What was the next medicinal step?
A   sitagliptin
B   rosiglitazone
C   a biguanide
D   a sulphonylurea
E   insulin

316 Which of the following is the most sensitive in making the diagnosis of early left heart failure in an elderly woman with a BMI = 32 kg/m²?
A   basal crepitations + raised JVP
B   plasma blood urea rise
C   raised concentration of serum creatinine
D   left ventricular echocardiogram
E   pro-B natriuretic peptide assay

317 When a patient with dementia is admitted to hospital, which of the following management strategies is less desirable than others?
A   one-to-one nursing
B   good lighting
C   single room
D   neuroleptics if needed
E   benzodiazepines if needed

318 An 81-year-old woman developed a tender scalp, jaw claudication, malaise and amaurosis fugax over a weekend. On Monday blood tests showed an anaemia, an eGFR of 35 and a CRP of 190. Her GP began oral prednisolone 60 mg that day. The following morning all features had departed and the CRP had fallen to 35.

What was the next step?
A do nothing further
B a myeloma screen
C ask for an urgent temporal artery biopsy
D arrange for a cancer protocol CT of thorax and abdomen
E investigate the anaemia

319 Despite good compliance it proved difficult to gain control of the hypertension of 76-year-old Robert Platt. Medication: perindopril 8 mg and amlodipine 10 mg.

Examination: well; BP 155/107; grade III hypertensive retinopathy; CXR: enlarged left ventricle.

What, according to the British Hypertension Society and NICE recommendations, should have been the next suitable step?
A add doxazosin
B add labetalol
C add hydralazine
D add candesartan
E add α methyl dopa

320 A patient with Diogenes syndrome (see Question 68) recovered quickly from a urinary infection – she had needed a hospital admission for management. Her home was infested with vermin enjoying the rotten food and half-eaten ready-prepared meals. The smell in her home was atrocious. The woman thought she was a little untidy and firmly refused any help. Many full bottles and blister packs of unused lithium carbonate were found.

What was the best management?
A to use the authority of the National Assistance Act 1948, Section 47 to rehouse the woman
B apply the 1961 Public Health Act to have the house emptied, cleaned and fumigated.
C assume the patient had capacity and let her continue living without change
D assess her capacity to make serious decisions
E reinstate the lithium therapy

321 Aged 70, Mrs Helen O Wills gave up smoking. Over the next 6 years her MBI rose from 26 to 33 kg/m². Latterly she woke at night with parathesiae in both hands. After several months she found that if she dangled her hands out of bed or shook them, the tingling almost ceased.

What was the most likely diagnosis?
A hypothyroidism
B median neuropathy
C hypocalcaemia
D obstructive sleep apnoea
E ulna neuropathy

322 A previously healthy man of 79 years died of cardiogenic shock. His younger brother developed repeated substernal 'feelings' and 'palpitations'. His company funded a BUPA assessment.

Examination: BMI 26.4; SR; daytime average BP profile 128/84; no cardiovascular signs.

Investigations: ECG; CXR; ECHO; ETT and adenosine stress isotopic tracer myocardial imaging: all normal. A 96-hour ECG was reported.

Which of the following was of clinical importance?
A heart rate of 38–42 whilst asleep overnight
B 25 periods of 4–6 second bursts of supraventricular tachycardia
C intermittent RBBB associated with a Mobitz type II
D a total of 874 ventricular ectopic beats
E 1100 atrial ectopics

323 Five years after quitting a 50-year nicotine addiction at the age of 70 years, Brian Fagg had an extensive anterior segment elevation myocardial infarction (STEMI). His hospital stay extended because of an infective exacerbation of his COAD. The day before the planned discharge, he was commenced on bisoprolol 1.25 mg.

What was the probable consequence of this action?
A acute bronchospasm
B a long-term reduction in his statistical mortality
C a heart rate of about 40 BPM
D a lasting fall in his FEV_1 of 30–35%
E Raynaud's phenomenon in winter

324 From the ABCD2 scoring system, what is the risk of an ischaemic stroke after a TIA in a 75-year-old person having had an isolated speech disturbance for 30 minutes. BP 150/95; HbA_{1c}: 6.0% (42).

A minor
B low
C medium
D high
E critical

325 The police brought an octogenarian to an A & E department because she had been found in her nightdress waiting at a disused bus stop at 2.30 a.m. A neighbour thought that she might have been 'off colour' for the previous few days.

Examination: disorientated in time and place, asking for her mother 'to take me home'. No other obvious physical signs.

Investigations:

urine dip:	awaited
CXR/AXR/ECG:	'nil acute' (medical registrar)
wbc	12.6 with 85% polymorphonuclears
CRP	134
albumin	34
AP	720 (< 300)
γGT	200 (< 50)
bilirubin	17

What was the most likely cause of her condition?
A urinary tract infection
B biliary sepsis
C frontal lobe stroke
D viral encephalitis
E secret alcoholism

326 Of the 'greying population', the 'older old' (> 85-year-olds) are increasing in numbers at the fastest rate. Which of the following is not a factor contributing to this extra longevity?
A better management of degenerative diseases
B enhanced perinatal services
C reduction in tenement housing
D vaccinations and antibiotics
E application of gerontological studies

327 An octogenarian gradually developed anterior bowing of both tibiae. They ached and felt warm.

Investigations:

CRP	8
Ca^{2+}	2.2
urate	235
ALT	44
AP	878
x-rays:	cotton wool thickening of calvarium
tibiae:	distortion of bone substance with pseudofractures

What was the diagnosis?
A   Bowen's disease
B   osteosclerosis
C   Paget's disease
D   osteomalacia
E   Marfan's syndrome

328 A 75-year-old woman was brought to her GP because of fever, dysuria and dehydration. There was some deterioration in renal function from a previously stable eGFR of 40. She took bisoprolol, warfarin, furosemide and a statin.

Examination: pulse irregular at 127; bi-basal creps; BP 140/90.

Investigations: urine: white cells; blood and protein.

Of the following, which is the most rational step?
A   prescribe digoxin
B   prescribe paracetamol
C   prescribe trimethoprim
D   prescribe amoxicillin
E   prescribe diltiazem

329 Angela Able, a previously healthy woman of 81 years, developed atrial fibrillation (AF) with a few days of dysphasia. A β-blocker controlled the ventricular rate to the region of 60–80 BPM. Echocardiography: mild aortic stenosis; right and left ejection fractions: preserved; TSH: 2.1.

Regarding anticoagulation strategies, which of the following was most suitable?
A paroxysmal AF is a weakish indication for warfarin
B aspirin is sufficient for a woman of that age – risk reduction about 50% (95% CL 40–70)
C warfarin + aspirin give greater protection
D the INR target range should be in the region of 2.5–3.5
E adequate warfarinisation confers a relative risk reduction of 70% (95% CL 50–80) and an absolute stroke reduction of 1.5 to 4.5%

330 Mrs Small-Puddle, a lady of uncertain seniority, became very tired because of invariable nocturia × 4–6. Her long-term medicines: thiazide, statin, aspirin with nocturnal TCA.

Which of the following was a potentially useful stratagem?
A a loop diuretic 5 hours before going to bed
B stop the thiazide
C stop the TCA
D try DDAVP
E try taking the thiazide dose in the early evening

331 When a person who had a right hemiplegia smiled, the left side of his mouth drooped.

The single lesion was where?
A right side of the brain stem
B left side of the brain stem
C cervical spine
D right motor cortex
E left motor cortex

332 Dorothy Jones (DOB 03/03/1933) was found slumped forward over a table in her day hospital. Her pulse was regular but there were pauses lasting up to 8 seconds.

Rhythm strip: normal PQRST activity but sinus pauses of up to 9 seconds

What was the diagnosis?
A intermittent complete heart block
B sinus arrhythmia
C transient ischaemic attack
D ventricular ectopic beats with compensatory pauses
E sick sinus syndrome

333 Na$^+$ 129; K$^+$ 2.4; random glucose 9.9; urate 420.

Which of the following drugs is likely to be implicated from the above data gathered from a woman of 83 years?
A citalopram
B azathioprine
C chlortalidone
D carbamazepine
E furosemide

334 The following features became available from a 74-year-old man who developed a persistent ulcer of his right 1st metatarsophalangeal joint.

Examination: ulcer: 12 mm lesion with serpiginous periphery; sensory-motor neuropathy; absent ankle jerks; proliferative retinopathy.

Investigations:

ulcer swabs:	commensal skin flora
CRP	50–80
eGFR	37
HbA$_{1c}$	9 (75)
x-ray of m-p joint:	no features of osteomyelitis
APBI:	normal

After 10 days of IV flucloxacillin and daily dressings, there was no healing of the ulcer.

What then was the most appropriate next step?
A CT of foot
B MRI of foot
C arteriogram of foot
D ^{18}fluoro-deoxy-glucose PET scan (^{18}FDG-PET scan)
E isotope bone scan

335 Considering the elderly colon: which one is wrong?
A constipation with overflow is often found
B constipation may present with vomiting
C endocrine diseases spare the large gut
D there is an increase in colonic fungi
E drug-induced colonic dysfunction is common

336 Which of the following is not a cause of onycholysis?
A MRSA sepsis
B psoriasis
C hyperthyroidism
D nail trauma
E psoralens

337 A 74-year-old man was sent up to a 'hot case' geriatric clinic on account of a symptomatic sitting to standing postural BP fall of 24/5 mm Hg.

Medicines: metformin, perindopril, amlodipine, simvastatin and aspirin.

Investigations:

creatinine	100
base line cortisol	129
post-Synacthen cortisol	670
HbA$_{1c}$	7.5 (59)

Which of the following would have been the least sensible action?
A stop amlodipine
B stop the ACEI
C prescribe midodrine
D measure adrenal antibodies
E apply TED stockings

338 The increasing age and number of first-world elderly populations, the substantial NHS and social care costs, the expansion of residential, nursing and specialist care homes together with models of chronic disease management have led to?
A an increase in numbers of consultant geriatricians
B better day hospital facilities
C greater media attention to hospital care associated with the care of elderly
D additional NICE guidelines issued
E a change in cases of prostatic carcinoma

339 Wm Flowerdew an 80-year-old gardener became 'fed up' with his invariable nocturia of × 5–7. He was never confident of complete voiding and since retiring daytime frequency was a nuisance – 'I miss them bushes'.

Examination: Digital Rectal Examination (DRE): normal size and constituency of prostate, empty rectum; BP 140/77; considerable OA of large joints and hands.

Investigations:

eGFR	54
PSA	3.7 (post-DRE)
glucose	6.0

What was the next single best managerial step?
A measure urine flow rate
B measure post-voiding residual volume
C send a MSU
D ultrasound imaging of prostate and trigone
E review of his medication

340 Over a weekend, a 74-year-old nursing home resident developed severe pain in and around her left eye. She felt poorly, nauseated and vomited her analgesic tablets. Coloured haloes were seen around lights. At an ED the signs were:

red conjunctiva
reduced visual acuity in the left eye
a fixed dilated pupil

What was the single diagnostic test needed?
A CT of brain structures
B temporal artery biopsy
C visual fields measurement
D tonometry
E conjunctival swab before antibiotics

341 Whilst visiting for chest pain, a 72-year-old chap collapsed in his GP's surgery. An ECG showed an evolving anterior STEMI with a sinus rate of 40 BPM.

Examination: in severe pain; cold and sweating; BP 85/50.

Apart from dialling 999, what first needs to be done?
A IV atropine
B IM morphia
C SC heparin
D GTN spray
E tablet of aspirin

342 A niece described her unmarried uncle's pre-morbid behaviour as kind, caring and placid, but over the latter 7 years he had gradually become impulsive and obnoxious. She was sure that his decline had been of insidious onset and then gradually progressed.

During some weeks of inpatient psychiatric stay it was possible to clarify that there had been a decline in social and interpersonal conduct. He was emotionally blunted, having lost insight 5 years previously.

Family history: his father and much older brother had died in a 'mental place' outside Calgary. An uncle had perished of motor neurone disease.

Investigation:

MMSE:	30/30
ACE R:	82/100 (reduction in verbal fluency)
FLAIR weighted MRI:	under perfusion of both frontal lobes
Psychological probes:	'difficult and challenging man showing evidence of perseveration and disinhibition'.

What was the diagnosis?
A AD
B localised vascular dementia
C fronto-temporal dementia
D Pick's disease
E Lewy Body disease

343 In hospitalised people, which of the following is associated with a low risk of the development of nosocomial pneumonia?
A esomeprazole
B ranitidine
C sucralfate
D famotidine
E pantoprazole

344 Which of the following suggestions about guidelines is correct?
A to be followed closely to avoid medical and nursing controversy
B to help avoid the delivery of substandard care
C to help reduce escalating NHS costs
D the best suggestions come from the DoH
E useful to help dodge lawyer's intrusions

345 Severe generalised OA in an overweight nonagenarian led to the development of pressure damage to skin over an ischium. The dermis was necrotic but deeper structures remained intact.

What was the correct treatment of the ulcer?
A ask a surgeon to debride the defect
B apply moist dressings, allow to dry and change at 48-hour intervals
C apply moist dressings, keep them moist and change them at 24-hour intervals
D use topical fusidic acid-impregnated daily dressings
E request debridement and pinch-skin grafts

346 Regarding donepezil, galantamine and rivastigmine: which of the following is or are correct?
A they function within weeks of beginning treatment
B about 50% of AD dementing patients will show improvement
C improvement is reliably recognised by a spouse or carer
D best started when the MMSE is about 25/30
E those who respond are more alert

347 A 75-year-old right-handed diabetic was brought to an ED because he had been 'talking strangely'. Mr Boxgrove understood requests and instructions, but enunciated words with difficulty and slowly. Sentences were shortened due to the non-use of prepositions and articles. Words that could be understood were appropriate for the sentence in which they were used.

Where was the lesion?
A right frontal lobe
B left frontal lobe
C right parietal lobe
D left parietal lobe
E corpus callosum

348 A 92-year-old man who lived alone with minimal external help developed an unpleasant lower respiratory tract infection. On admission: CURB-65 score = 5. Six weeks later, whilst improving, he was just able to transfer alone and just able to pass the kitchen test but would not have been able to complete his daily newspaper trip of 250 m. His home toilet was on the upper story of his house. His children were believed to be in the wine business in Chile.

His MDT decided that the best next step was to be:
A to return him to his two-story house with a commode
B to set him up in a residential home
C to find a rehabilitation ward for 8 weeks
D to see about selling his house for residential funds
E to seek a warden-controlled sheltered accommodation facility

349 Despite appropriate doses of perindopril, furosemide and spirolactone, Mrs LV Few's congestive heart failure progressed. Her COPD was adequately controlled with tiotropium, as was her T1DM.

Examination: Class IV New York dyspnoea; BP 114/74; SR, 98 BPM.

Investigations:

LVEF	circa 20%
eGFR	37
HbA$_{1c}$	7.1 (54)
CXR:	dilated left ventricle; Kerley B lines.

She was given a selective β-blocker.

What was her likely outlook?
A statistically an extension of her life
B a transient worsening of her COPD
C a probable persistent worsening of her COPD
D an altered appreciation of hypoglycaemia
E an increased statistical chance of hospital admissions

350 The following results were obtained from a frail, bed-bound, wasted 92-year-old man, resident in an EMI unit.

MMSE:	11/30
Hb	7.7
MCV	75

blood film: hypochromic, microcytic red cells

Which of the following statements constituted the most sensible course?

A request virtual colonoscopy
B ask for a sigmoidoscopy
C do nothing
D prescribe 3 months of iron
E transfuse 2 units of blood

Answers 1–350

1 A

The substantially raised MCV, mild anaemia, thrombocytopenia and leuco-poenia, all fit with an 'early' (pre-symptomatic) B_{12} deficiency state. The blood film showed macrocytes – the source of the raised MCV and hyper-segmented neutrophil white cells – 'PA polys'. The serum concentration of B_{12} was sub-normal. While the finding of serum antibodies against intrinsic factor (present in 60% of cases) aids the diagnosis, the diagnosis depends upon an infranormal serum B_{12} concentration, the characteristic blood film and response to replacement therapy.

2 A

Loss of consciousness results from impairment of the vertobasilar territory circulation, which of itself is an infrequent TIA defining event. Fainting, hypoglycaemia, partial seizures and hyperventilation are principal conditions which should present in the differential diagnosis of loss of consciousness.

B to E are all typical TIA features.

see McArthur KS *et al.*, Diagnosis and management of TIAs and ischaemic stroke in the acute phase. *BMJ*. 2011; **342**: 812–7.

3 E

Drugs A to C have potential bladder benefits but, without expanding the history, making an examination and perhaps performing some investigations, a sensible decision cannot be made. Note that the terms anticholinergic and antimuscarinic are synonymous, with anticholinergic being the preferred term. Additionally a 5α-reductase inhibitor has no therapeutic place in the treatment of a woman.

see Marinkovic SP. The management of overactive bladder syndrome. *BMJ*. 2012; **344**: 38–44.

4 C

Fifty to 60% of all pelvic fractures involve two rami on the same side. An inferior ramus fracture alone is found in about 20% and other patterns to lesser extents.

5   C

An elderly person in an institutional environment taking a diet different from their usual is very prone to become constipated. Faecal stagnation develops gradually before becoming symptomatic. Constipation leading to vomiting is not an infrequent reason for acute hospital admission. The condition has to be differentiated from intestinal obstruction, which is much less frequent.

6   E

Mr Green had the restless legs syndrome (Eckbom's syndrome; Swedish neurologist). This responds to dopamine agonists: ropinirole is usually used.

The eye changes and absence of deep tendon reflexes are normal features in a number of elderly people. They had no bearing on Mrs Green's disturbed sleep.

7   C

Mr Best had an arterial ulcer. It was essential to maintain or enhance the blood supply to the foot. A compression bandage might have worsened the already borderline foot perfusion and should not be used. Before applying a bandage it is essential to demonstrate that the ankle:brachial pressure index is > 0.9.

8   D

Insulin glargine has activity for over 24 hours. If the patient delays or misses a meal she is at risk of hypoglycaemia and confusion. A BM reading pre-breakfast has no bearing on what may occur later in the day. More data was required.

9   C

Isaacs (1992) characterised the non-specific presentational features of illness in the elderly by the following: Immobility, Instability, Incontinence and Intellectual Impairment. 'They have in common the qualities of: multiple causation, chronic course, deprivation of independence and no simple cure.' Some add iatrogenic illness to the 'four giants'.

Isaacs B. *The Challenge of Geriatric Medicine*. Oxford: Oxford Medical Publications; 1992.

10   B

A pharyngeal pouch causes local symptoms including regurgitation of saliva and food but not iron deficiency. Lack of compliance is the usual reason for failure to respond to iron therapy. Nevertheless coeliac disease (A) and gut bleeds (E) are common explanations for failure of iron tablets. Note that while the blood films of patients with thalassaemia trait show microcytic hypochromic red cells, such people are not iron deficient and iron is not needed (see Answer 39).

11 E

Uterine prolapse is often asymptomatic but some women experience an intra-vaginal fullness or heaviness. A to D are accepted causes of pruritus vulvae.

12 E

This 75-year-old-man had developed presbycusis (age-related hearing loss – sensorineural degeneration). Typical symptoms are those outlined in the vignette which may lead to a person withdrawing from social activities with resulting isolation. Hearing aids help some. Understanding of conversation is helped by low-pitched speech in a quiet environment. Lip reading may be useful. The defects in hearing affect both sensory peripheral (cochlea) and central (neuronal) pathways.

13 B

An informal carer is usually a family member or relative who is not formally employed to provide help. Much state funding is unclaimed due to ignorance of these non-means-tested benefits. The AA cannot be claimed retrospectively.

Most carers are in the 55+ age band and are at risk of chronic stress-related illness and impaired health. Carers in their teens are at risk of social, educational and mental health difficulties.

see Cameron ID, Aggar C, Robinson AL, Kurrie SE. Assessing and helping carers of older people. *BMJ*. 2011; **343**: 630–3.

14 A

Suggestions B to E indicate the need for specialist help. A patient diagnosed with colorectal cancer below the age of 45 years has some form of familial malignancy. Older patients such as Flo Smith develop the sporadic form of bowel cancer for which there is no familial association.

15 E

The largest percentage growth in population is in men and women aged > 85 years of age. The economics (including the 'gray' £) and political strength of people in their latter quarter of life will continue to grow as will their health needs.

see Evans JG. Geriatrics. *Clin Med*. 2011; **11**: 166–9.

16 B

The vignette describes a patient with a gradual onset of temporal arteritis (giant cell arteritis) and separates it from the other suggested conditions. Matters are urgent: amaurosis fugax often precedes permanent visual loss.

17 D

The patient was considered to have an overactive thyroid from the history and findings. TSH: 9.8.

18 B

The decision to begin what will be lifelong treatment is ideally made jointly between the informed patient and his doctor. It is held that early treatment potentially improves long-term motor outcomes. Useful patient information is available from www.parkinsonsdisease.org.

see Grosset DG, MacPhee GJA, Nairn M. Diagnosis and pharmacological management of Parkinson's disease. *BMJ*. 2010; **340**: 206–9.

19 C

This feature is essential to the diagnosis of fibromyalgia. A, B, D and E are incorrect.

20 E

It has become most important to be able to detect age-related macular degeneration early because blindness can be prevented by intravitreal injections of monoclonal vascular endothelial growth factor inhibitor. Up to 30% of over 75s may have early disease and 7% late disease. Distortion of central vision necessitates urgent specialist analysis.

see Chakravarty U, Evans J, Rosenfield PI. Age related macular degeneration. *BMJ*. 2011; **340**: 526–30.

21 B

Sir Julian had postural hypotension and a very low MCV suggested iron deficiency anaemia. This, together with his substantial alcohol intake suggested an alcoholic gastritis from which low-grade bleeding had occurred. Endoscopy that afternoon at The London Clinic established the diagnosis of a haemorrhagic gastritis.

22 A

Women tend to fall more than men. A multidisciplinary team can sort out possible polypharmacy hazards, the use of sedatives, medical diseases, muscular weakness, balance and gait deficiencies, the wearing of spectacles and home-related environmental hazards. Any fall tends to increase the faller's disability, and lessen confidence in balance and mobility such that independent existence becomes impossible. A fractured femur has a 30-day mortality rate of 15–20%.

see Close JCT, Lord SR. Fall assessment in older people. *BMJ*. 2011; **343**: 579–82.

23 E

The diagnosis is suggested by the triad of slow intellectual loss, broad-based gait, unsteadiness and early incontinence. The diagnosis is made by CT brain imaging showing enlarged ventricles. Ventriculo-peritoneal shunting may arrest the decline.

24 B

The blood film in conjunction with the splenomegaly (site of the extramedullary haematopoiesis) and the inability to aspirate bone marrow ('dry tap'; marrow fibrosis) secure the diagnosis. The large red cells (MCV 105) were explained by the tear drop poikilocytes, which are larger than healthy red cells. The term 'leukoerythroblastic' is used when in the same blood film there are nucleated red and white cells.

25 A

By 6 months some 25% of ischaemic stroke (IS) patients will have died. About 50% of IS survivors have varying degrees of hemiparesis at 6 months post-acute event. About 15% of IS patients will have had a preceding TIA. Overall the figures are improving with the development of specific acute stroke facilities and the use of tissue plasminogen activator ≤3 hours after onset of the 'brain attack'.

see Wechsler LR. Intravenous thrombolytic therapy for acute ischaemic stroke. *New Engl J Med.* 2011; **364**: 2138–64.

26 C

This man had 'taken to the bottle' after his wife's death and his behaviour was more than his adult children were able to tolerate. Broken bones, bruises and scratches are common in alcoholics. The jaundice and raised alanine transferase indicated liver damage. The normal alkaline phosphatase implies no obstruction of bile drainage. The raised MCV 'fits' both liver disease and direct alcohol toxicity. The ferritin, raised at 505, was an acute phase reactant.

27 B

The thoracic spine is affected in approximately 70% of cases and the lumbar in 20%. Diffuse metastatic compression is very uncommon. Of the whole skeleton the spinal column is the commonest site for metastases. Cord compression affects 5–10%. The most common primary tumours are breast, prostate and lung.

28 C

Diabetic nephropathy tops the list. In some patients it is a preventable cause of developing Stage V chronic kidney disease (CKD V; eGFR ≤ 15 ml/minute/1.75 m^2 body surface area).

29 E

It is a common error to prescribe allopurinol at a daily dose of 300 mg. This dose in elderly people is too high for routine purposes and is associated with an increased incidence of side-effects – rash and hypersensitivity reactions. For most older patients, the correct dose of allopurinol is 100 mg daily. This is particularly true in renal failure (common in the elderly) and in chronic liver disease.

see Lipworth W. Suboptimal prescribing: chronic gout. *BMJ*. 2011; **343**: 1193–5.

30 B

Sweating and tachycardia are well-recognised consequences of tricyclic anti-depressant treatment and reverse upon stopping the drug.

31 D

The persistent perception of musical or other understandable sounds suggests a psychiatric or neurological condition. It is not a feature of tinnitus. High doses of aspirin or furosemide may cause a reversible tinnitus.

32 B

The commonest is a basal cell carcinoma (BCC). It grows slowly, is locally invasive ('rodent ulcer') and is found more frequently in people with fair skins after chronic sun exposure. The majority develop on the lower lid. A BCC begins as a nodule which very slowly enlarges, leaving a central depression – the 'rolled edge'. The tumour usually has telangiectatic vessels on the surface.

33 E

H pylori serology may remain positive for years after complete eradication of the gastric infestation. Serological measurements have no part to play in assessing treatment. Some antibodies persist lifelong after clearing of an initial infection (infectious mononucleosis, for example).

see Braden B. Diagnosis of *H pylori* infection. *BMJ*. 2012; **344**: 44–6

34 E

Primary open-angle glaucoma is asymptomatic until impairment in vision is noted. The macular is spared, leading to tunnel vision. The less common acute angle-closure glaucoma, where there is a rapid increase in intraocular pressure, causes a painful red eye, blurred vision and haloes. Carbonic anhydrase inhibitors – acetazolamide and dorzolamide may lead to an acute metabolic acidosis if used in renal impairment.

35 E

The reduced plasma sodium had been present for years in a healthy elderly female. Thus 'if it ain't broke, don't fix it' applies. And don't induce unnecessary anxiety in the patient about an asymptomatic, unimportant plasma sodium assay result or waste time and money on unnecessary investigations.

36 A

The presence of leucocyte esterase is a marker for pyuria and urine culture is indicated. A positive nitrite test would suggest the presence of a coliform.

From the information presented, no reliable deduction as to the level of renal function can be made. The PSA might be raised if the school mistress had had a metastasised breast carcinoma.

37 C

The signs of fracture of femoral neck and hip replacement may be identical. A person with a fractured hip may be able to walk. An operation is the treatment of choice for all except those who have substantial co-morbidities. The 30-day mortality following surgery is 15–20%. Traction has a very considerable morbidity and mortality. The cost to the State of a fractured femur is conservatively priced at £15k (2010 prices).

38 D

While an inability to perform adequately any of the necessities of everyday living may have mental consequences, reduced mood and altered thinking is not an ADL.

39 E

The laboratory data are typical figures for thalassaemia trait – very low MCV, MCHC with raised red blood cell count – which is common in Cyprus. The MCV is too low for an iron deficiency anaemia or anaemia of chronic disease (75–80; 75–82, respectively) and blood ferritin concentration is within the reference range. Thalassaemia trait is an asymptomatic harmless abnormality inherited as an autosomal recessive. Thalassaemias have a geographical distribution stretching from Portugal across the Mediterranean, the Middle East, India and Malaysia to the Far East.

40 C

An excess production of parathyroid hormone, usually from a single adenoma is the most common cause of hypercalcaemia in 80% of elderly people. The incidence of primary hyperparathyroidism peaks in the 7th decade; most cases occur in women. The condition is usually detected on routine calcium assay in asymptomatic people. Gone are the days of 'bones, stones and abdominal groans' as (late) presentational features.

see Marcocci C, Cetani F. Primary hyperparathyroidism. *New Engl J Med.* 2011; **365**: 2389–97.

41 B

Irene Felty had advanced rheumatoid arthritis with typical hand features. Using a toilet seat of standard height was painful and difficult. The raised seat eased sitting and the pain of regaining standing.

Heberden's nodes are characteristic of osteoarthritis and not a feature of pure rheumatoid arthritis. The principal rheumatological association with HLA B27 is ankylosing spondylitis. Miss Felty did not have the strength of grip to brake a rollator: her instability would worsen. The forearm rests of a gutter frame are helpful for people with impaired hand or wrist function.

42 B

Angiotensin converting enzyme inhibitors (ACEI) and angiotensin II receptor blockers (ARB) do not produce a useful fall in blood pressure in two groups of hypertensives:

a Those over the age of 55 years; and
b Black people of African or Caribbean family origin.

Such drugs should not be used for these people because the therapeutic effect is marginal, since the two groups have low tissue concentrations of angiotensin; there is therefore little for an ACEI or ARB to inhibit and thus reduce the blood pressure.

43 E

The blood sample was not treated correctly from being drawn to assay. Kept overnight at ambient temperatures, potassium would have extruded from erythrocytes, leading to a falsely elevated plasma concentration. If there is to be delay in the transport of blood to a laboratory for potassium assay, the sample should either be discarded or centrifuged and serum separated from cells. In the vignette with an eGFR of 35, an endogenous hyperkalaemia would not be expected because at that level of renal function potassium excretion is not usually reduced.

44 E

Features A to D are all correct. By the age of 80 years, AD has a prevalence of 15–50%. Amyloid deposition in the brain may be demonstrated from the fifties onwards. The characteristic histopathology includes extracellular plaques containing fibrillary amyloid β peptides and intracellular neurofibrillary tangles of hyperphosphorylated (insoluble) τ protein.

Alzheimer is believed to have died (aged 51) of renal failure as a consequence of proliferative glomerulonephritis secondary to subacute bacterial endocarditis.

see Harwood RH. Dementia for hospital physicians. *Clin Med.* 2012; **12**: 35–9.

45 D

Joan would remain secure in the family-owned home for as long as she wished. Some of their joint income would be lost because a proportion of Derby's state pension would be diverted to meet his upkeep. All of his savings above £23 250 would be used for his maintenance but £23 250 would have remained for his exclusive use. It is estimated that the annual cost to the British State for elderly care services is, at 2011 prices, £2.65 billion.

This is the position in early 2012 but funding rates are reviewed annually and may change.

see Henwood M. Review of funding for social care in England. *BMJ*. 2011; **343**: 5

46 D

Onycholysis (the painless loosening of the nail from the nail bed) is often present, which permits fungal infection. Malnutrition and diabetes may contribute to the establishment and persistence of Candida sp. Koilonychia usually reflects an iron deficiency with or without anaemia.

47 E

The two commas sign is found when a person who does not have Parkinson's disease (PD) is studied by axial single photon emission computed tomography (SPECT) scanning. In PD dopaminergic cells in the substantia nigra degenerate. Consequently the radiolabelled ligand localises less well. In health a SPECT scan images the substantia nigra as comma shapes. Distorted or reduced comma shapes correspond to the presence of less dopamine transporter.

Thus if two well-defined commas are imaged on a SPECT scan the patient does not have PD.

A The Kerley B (septal) line is a chest x-ray feature – comprising distended interlobular lymphatics at right angles to the pleural surface as seen in left ventricular failure and mitral stenosis.

B Colonic carcinoma may infiltrate the bowel wall circumferentially, leading to irregular luminal narrowing: the apple core sign, found at barium enema examination.

C The pepper pot skull is the description of multiple lytic lesions of the cranial vault in multiple myeloma.

D Honeycomb lung is a high resolution CT appearance of the lungs – a generalised reticular pattern – and is a late feature of some chronic lung diseases.

see Breen DP, Rowe JB, Barker RA. Role of brain imaging in early parkinsonism. *BMJ*. 2011; **342**: 495–8.

48 E

Nail pitting may be seen in psoriasis; it is not sub-nutritionally induced. A to D are correct. Ankle jerks are absent in about 20% of healthy elderly people, which has no pathological importance.

49 A

The Waterlow score of pressure scoring has four stages. Stage 1: non-blanching erythema of intact skin; 2: partial thickness skin loss; 3: full-thickness skin loss through fat down to the depth of the underlying facia; 4: full-thickness loss to the depth of muscle, tendon or bone.

Rivermead is a mobility index; the Gleason score is used to quantify the degree of cellular aggressiveness of carcinoma of the prostate; the Hamilton score is a scale for grading depression and the Barthel index quantifies a patient's daily activities.

50 E

At 80% the oxygen saturation is low despite a high inspired oxygen concentration (FiO_2). A low saturation (and PaO_2) favours a large proximally lodged embolus. The D-dimer assay was irrelevant – Miss Fern had had an operation with tissue damage and blood spilling only three days before blood was sampled for D-dimer assay. An assay for D-dimer is only of value if the result is within the reference range. However high an abnormal result, it does not necessarily indicate the presence of a pulmonary embolus. A positive result reflects a clot somewhere, but has no localising quality.

51 D

Miss Brody had a reactive depression as a consequence of Crème's death and her social losses.

see Rodda J, Walker Z, Carter J. Depression in older adults. *BMJ*. 2011; **343**: 683–7.

52 C

From the age of 14 this man had had 51 years of exposure to coal dust and had developed progressive massive fibrosis (PMF; complicated mineworker's pneumoconiosis). Chest x-rays showed irregular opacities in the upper lobes with background nodular shadowing. The opacities may cavitate liberating black material (melanoptysis). PMF is a compensable industrial disease.

53 C

The patient's best interests are paramount, including medical, physical, spiritual, social and all other factors relevant to his or her welfare. The converse is true regarding A, C, D and E. The LCP should be reviewed regularly, and is applicable to a dying person of any age to meet his or her differing needs. Age and diagnosis have little direct bearing on the LCP-delivered care.

54 B

This is a prospective study, the cohort being the 300 patients trying the new calcium tablet. Once selected the cohort is then fixed to the final outcome of the study – whether continuing to take the new preparation or not.

55 E

Section 5(2) empowers a doctor to detain a person for a maximum of 72 hours under the authority of a responsible physician. Such a doctor is usually the consultant or his nominated deputy. Detention may be in a general or psychiatric hospital while the patient's mental health is assessed.

The Mental Health Acts 1983 and 2007 are complex and advice from a psychogeriatrician should be taken before the 72 hours expire.

56 A

The converse is true; a person's impairment tends to induce unthinking discrimination for the reason that the impaired are 'different' and that it is 'their fault'. Such discrimination takes many forms as B to E indicate. Previously entrenched opposing opinions between medical and social models are moving to a neutral 'working together' model.

57 B

The use of bupropion, a dopamine reuptake inhibitor, doubles the success rate of smoking cessation. It is contraindicated in epileptics. Varenicline is also used. It is a partial nicotine agonist and is more effective than bupropion. Nevertheless, the quit rate at one year is only 20%.

58 B

The history and weight data show that Ken Pound had retained fluid – some of it intrapulmonary. As previously advised, he doubled the dose of furosemide and continued to record his daily weight. If weight (and therefore fluid) loss were not to occur he would have needed medical help. A week later, Mr Pound had lost 4 kg and his dyspnoea largely resolved.

Changing the aldosterone antagonist, eplerenone, would have given no advantage. To swap furosemide for an equipotent bumetanide dose would have been illogical. If either furosemide or bumetanide are 'not working', swapping one equipotent dose to the other will gain no advantage.

59 C

Painful, unbidden reminders of very traumatic events (military or civilian), even after 50 years, is very compatible with, and suggestive of, post-traumatic stress disorder. A psychiatrist, preferably with a military background, is essential. There are a number of charities who specialise in helping afflicted ex-military personnel.

see Gabriel R, Leigh AN. PTSD following military combat or peace keeping. *BMJ*. 2002; **324**: 340–1.

60 A

Anaemia – normochromic, normocytic (both MCV and MCHC within their reference ranges) – is present in about 75% of myeloma patients at diagnosis. The anaemia is explained by bone marrow infiltration by plasma cells or renal dysfunction or both.

61 D

A DNAR directive may be cancelled by a specialist registrar (ST3 or above), a GP partner or salaried GP or hospital consultant. An entry should be made in the clinical records and nursing staff informed.

The converse is true of the statements A, B, C and E.

see Slouther A-M. Medical futility and DNR orders. *Clin Ethics.* 2006; **1**: 18–20.

62 D

The history, BMI and investigational findings of Mr Hearty (Class II obesity) exactly fit the diagnosis of non-alcoholic fatty liver disease (NAFLD), which is a state of benign fatty liver infiltration (hepatic steatosis). A proportion of these people progress to inflammation, cirrhosis and portal hypertension – end-stage non-alcoholic steatohepatitis (NASH). It is likely that NASH is or will become the most common cause of end-stage liver disease in developed countries.

see Day CP. Non-alcoholic fatty liver disease. *Clin Med.* 2011; **11**: 176–8.

63 E

All suggestions A to E are viable but the estimated glomerular filtration rate (eGFR) as calculated by the MDRD equation is the best so far devised. All chemical pathology departments should now report renal function as serum creatinine and eGFR in ml/minute/1.73 m^2.

  A serum creatinine alone requires considerable experience to interpret adequately
  B creatinine clearance is acceptable but usually inaccurate because urine collection and timing of blood sampling often invalidate the result to an unknown, unknowable degree.
  C the CG formula has now been superseded by the MDRD calculation which is performed by the laboratory computer
  D the CKD classification of renal function can lead to misclassification and misunderstanding of the degree of renal failure. It is simplest to avoid the risk of obfuscation and not use the CKD system. The eGFR is simpler and better.

Knowledge of renal function is more important in elderly patients than other branches of general medicine because of frequent renal functional impairment which may be relevant to drug dosage.

64 D

Both thiazides and SSRIs are well known to induce hyponatraemia. Either could have been operative in Mr Salt; both should have been withdrawn.

Also, it was not good practice to make the two diagnoses at the same time because the stress of depression might well have elevated a normal blood pressure. A decision to treat an elevated BP should be made very infrequently at the first clinical encounter.

65 C

Like stars, false teeth should come out at night. Statements A, B, D, E are correct.

The continuous wearing of dentures positively correlates with chronic oral disease, particularly if the dentures are ill-fitting. Relieving the mouth by removal of dentures for the night allows normal mucosal auto-hygiene to occur and for denture disinfection by overnight storage in a cold 1% sodium hypochlorite solution.

Edentulism tends to be found in the elderly of less affluent social backgrounds.

66 C

Gliclazide has no sodium or water-retaining properties and is therefore the most appropriate choice in the context of Q 66.

67 C

Furosemide is needed for symptom control by enhancing sodium and water excretion. ACEI drugs have been shown to reduce heart failure mortality. A thiazide has no place. Spironolactone also reduces heart failure deaths and is usually started with clearing of the oedema.

68 D

This is the Diogenes or squalor syndrome. Risk factors include an eccentric personality, social isolation, impaired vision or suffering a recent bereavement in a mildly demented or depressed elderly person. The individual is unwilling to reason or accept help.

69 A

The 'velcro-like' sounds, while not pathognomonic, are highly suggestive of pulmonary fibrosis.

70 C

Because there is a risk that a bleeding gastric ulcer may be malignant but cannot be biopsied at the acute phase, a repeat endoscopy to check ulcer status is always needed.

71 E

Answers A to D are correct. E is incorrect; free radicals are believed to be central to the pathophysiology of increasing age. The theory holds that when the production of reactive oxygen species exceeds antioxidant buffering mechanisms, there is damage to the sugar-phosphate DNA backbone. Nucleic acid repair becomes increasingly less efficient and eventually oxidative phosphorylation decreases so that reduced ATP production declines, leading to cell death.

72 B

Coliform bacteria (*E coli*, Klebsiella species and Enterobacter) reduce urinary nitrates to nitrites.

Cephalosporin treatment, unless there were special circumstances, would not be appropriate because of the risk of predisposing the patient to *Clostridium difficile* (CD) infestation. The organism is a gram positive spore-forming anaerobic bacterium; some 5% of healthy adults carry CD as part of their normal gut flora.

see Cormican M, Murphy AW, Vellinga A. Interpreting asymptomatic bacteria. *BMJ*. 2011; **343**: 364–7.

73 E

This is a typical case of Lewy Body disease (LBD). From apparent idiopathic Parkinson's disease (PD), there were rapid changes as shown by the development of hallucinations a few months from the first diagnosis. Response to dopamine diminished and there was early impairment of higher cerebral function. In PD, cognitive decline and dementia are late (years) features. Cognitive decline has to precede or occur within a year of the onset of motor findings for the clinical diagnosis of LBD to be made.

74 E

The official recommendation for the treatment (and prophylaxis) of osteoporosis is to supply calcium supplementation of the diet, a bisphosphonate to enhance osteoblastic calcium deposition and a vitamin D preparation to aid the absorption of calcium from the gut.

see Favus MJ. Bisphosphonates for osteoporosis. *New Engl J Med*. 2010; **363**: 2027–35.

75 A

Answers B and C were potentially useful courses, providing Poppy were to be in agreement. She had taken months to decide to travel to Zurich. Because Poppy had the mental capacity to weigh the pros and cons of her decision, her autonomous choice had to be respected.

The use of high-dose opiates to suppress pain might have indirectly been fatal. This passive euthanasia is legal if administered with good intent – the double effect principle. Such patient management should be discussed with the patient, relatives, senior doctors and a defence society before setting in place.

76 E

People with essential tremor are no more prone to constipation than a suitable control group. Alcohol and β-blockers damp down the tremor. There is often a positive family history; essential tremor is inherited as an autosomal dominant in about 50% of cases.

77 D

The ampicillin had displaced some of the albumin-bound warfarin, thereby increasing the amount of anticoagulant available to inhibit coagulation. Both warfarin and the penicillin should have been stopped. If there was no bleeding, vitamin K was not indicated because if used, subsequent warfarin doses would be difficult to judge for several weeks. Warfarin reduces the synthesis of prothrombin and coagulation factors VII, IX and X. In an emergency these components can be supplied via an infusion of prothrombin complex.

see Garcia D. Practical management of coagulopathy associated with warfarin. *BMJ*. 2011; **340**: 918–20

78 B

After 5 to 10 years of tyrosine kinase inhibitor treatment, the majority of patients with CML gradually transform to an accelerated phase. The remainder move abruptly to acute blastic transformation and have the sudden development of symptoms to match. The patient then has acute myeloid leukaemia and has to be treated accordingly.

79 D

Bradykinesia is considered to be a defining feature of Parkinson's disease. The tremor is of 4–6 Hz amplitude but asymmetrical; rigidity is accentuated by use of the contralateral limb; postural instability is a late feature.

80 E

The very slow heart rate was an idioventricular rhythm. It was not a sinus bradycardia because the P-waves were, while regular, independent of the ventricular (QRS) contractions. The atrial impulse was not crossing the atrioventricular node and therefore not activating the ventricles. A permanent pacemaker was required urgently.

81 C

The details in Question 81 fit total global amnesia most closely – the age of onset, duration of symptoms, ability to perform high-level activity (driving) and the sequelae are typical.

82 D

After application of a non-adherent dressing and being sure that the arterial supply to the leg is acceptable (normal range ankle brachial pressure index 1.0–1.3) the correct order of bandage application is 1, 2, 3 and 4.

83 D

Providing the FEV_1 was > 50% of predicted, a long-acting β_2 agonist (LABA; formoterol, salmeterol) would have been appropriate. If the FEV_1 was < 50% of predicted, then a LABA should have been combined with an inhaled corticosteroid in a combination inhaler.

see Drugs & Therap Bull. 2010; **48**: 74–7.

Wedzicha JA. Choice of bronchodilator therapy for patients with COPD. *New Eng J Med.* 2011; **364**: 1167–8.

Niewoehner DE. Outpatient Management of Severe COPD. *New Engl J Med.* 2011; **362**: 1407–16.

84 B

The VI cranial nerve (abducens) is the odd one out. It supplies the lateral rectus muscle, causing the eye to abduct: this causes diplopia upon looking to the affected side. An isolated VI palsy is often attributed to damage to the blood supply to the nerve (vasa nevorum) secondary to diabetes or hypertension. The microvascular damage usually clears completely within a few months. An isolated VI palsy may also be a false localising sign when there is raised intracranial pressure.

85 E

The shock delivered by a defibrillator is not insubstantial: it would be very distressing, inappropriate and constitute poor medical practice. The dyspnoea of COPD responds well to suitably judged doses of morphia. Cyclizine is best avoided in heart failure because it is pro-arrhythmic. Death from hyperkalaemia, per se, is painless. Conversely, over half of people with advanced multiple sclerosis experience different varieties of pain: opioids, adjuvant analgesics, anticonvulsants, antimuscarinics and baclofen are often required in different proportions and doses.

86 E

The history suggests a progressive left hemisphere lesion. Because a head injury preceded the onset of symptoms, the most likely diagnosis is subdural haematoma. Such haematomata are more common in people taking antiplatelet or anticoagulant drugs.

87 A

The description given fits the diagnosis of a seborrhoeic wart (basal cell papilloma). These lesions are benign and consist of a proliferation of basal keratinocytes. They are often multiple. Mrs Hay had hers treated by hyfrecation.

88 E

Urgent senior advice was essential. Valid binding advanced life refusal of life-sustaining treatment must be in writing, applicable to specific circumstances and must state that it is to apply even if life is threatened. The directive has to be signed and witnessed. The SHO had to discuss matters with his consultant and discuss the validity of the husband's representations. The unseen advanced directive could not have been taken as binding but was taken into account as the patient's prior wishes. The SHO and physician had to decide what was in the patient's best interest.

see General Medical Council. *Treatment and Care Towards the End of Life*. London: GMC; 2010.

Mental Capacity Act 2005 and the mental capacity code of practice (England & Wales only)

89 A

The sudden development of chest features in a person receiving enteral feeding is due to aspiration of feed until proved otherwise. The presence of a nasogastric tube does not protect a person from aspiration.

90 C

The calculation:	eye opening to pain	2
	incomprehensible speech	3
	localisation to pain	5
	total	10

No response for eye opening, speech or pain scores: 3.

see Teasdale G, Jennett B. Assessment of coma and impaired consciousness. A practical scale. *Lancet*. 1974; ii: 81–4.

91 E

Items A–D are independent risk factors for falling. Poor gait and impaired balance are late, not early features of Parkinson's disease. Should a patient apparently suffering from parkinsonism develop falls in the early months of the condition, the original diagnosis would very probably be incorrect. Many disparate factors may contribute to falls in the elderly.

see Close JCT, Lord SR. Fall assessment in older people. *BMJ*. 2011; **343**: 579–82.

92 A

The gold standard of the diagnosis of Alzheimer's dementia (AD) is brain histology (see Answer 44) which makes or denies the diagnosis. Brain biopsy is not a realistic procedure for a condition lacking adequate treatment. Nevertheless, brain histology diagnosis has the sensitivity of one. That is, there would be no false positives or negatives: the gold standard. The proponents of the new non-invasive test had to approach that degree of accuracy. With a high specificity a positive result means that AD is present. With a high sensitivity a negative result means that AD is absent. Thus both specificity and sensitivity have to score 1 (or 100%) to fulfil these rigorous criteria. Clinically the predication rates are the most relevant within a defined population. Very few tests are reliable in identifying both positive and negative features.

93 A

This woman had thyroiditis. In this condition the hyperthyroid state is transient. A β-blocker alone controls symptoms until the condition evolves into euthyroidism or hypothyroidism.

94 B

Cimetidine binds to microsomal cytochrome P450 and should be avoided in patients established on warfarin, phenytoin, valporate and theophylline – all frequently used in elderly people. Ranitidine does not have the P450 inhibitory property of cimetidine.

Elderly people are frequently subjected to polypharmacy (more than 4 drugs per day) and overall tolerate drugs less well than younger folk. The incidence of Types A and B adverse reactions is greater with increasing age. Thus, assuming H_2 blockade is required, the choice of ranitidine over cimetidine is a step towards safer drug deployment. Also, non-proprietary ranitidine tablets are cheaper than the cimetidine equivalent.

95 D

Only the diagnosis of Paget's disease of the nipple fits the described clinical features and treatment failures. In particular eczema is usually bilateral, does not have clear margins, fluctuates, may be moist and responds to topical steroids. The adage 'beware unilateral eczema' applies.

96 A

NICE guidelines state that in diabetics a new foot ulcer or skin colour alteration should be seen by experts within 24 hours of its recognition. Diabetic foot disease is a major cause of morbidity and is common. The morbidity and mortality increase in parallel with increasing age.

see Tam T *et al.* NICE guidelines on management of diabetic foot problems. *BMJ.* 2011; **342**: 702–3.

97 A

This old man had few pleasures left and the quality of his remaining months was more important than the duration. While drinking tea risked an inhalation pneumonitis, not to allow Mr Grey his favourite drink would be unkind, inappropriate and poor medical practice.

98 D

A 'no fall risk' comprises getting up from a seat, walking 3 m (10 ft), turning through 360° and then walking the 3 m back to the seat. All movements should be well co-ordinated and completed without any walking aid.

A fully mobile person will complete the test in < 10 seconds; < 20 is classed as mostly independent, 20–30 and > 30 seconds as variable or impaired, respectively.

99 E

Key features of delirium include an acute onset, fluctuation (hourly or daily) in cognition, inattention, distractibility, altered levels of consciousness and disorganised thinking. Recent memory is always affected, long-term memory to a lesser extent. Gradual worsening in cogitative decline is an essential feature of dementia. When a delirium clears, the person's memory returns to the pre-delirious level.

100 C

The study did not take place over time. A cross-sectional (point prevalence) study takes a 'snapshot' at the time, of different prescribing patterns in the 6 medical wards.

101 C

The data best fit hyperpyrexia secondary to sustained exogenous high ambient temperatures with substantial dehydration (Na^+ 152; albumin 75). Autoregulation had failed with the development of heat stroke. The mortality is > 50% in the elderly who present with depressed cerebral function. Elderly people behave as being relatively poikilothermic with weakened homeostasis.

102 B

Over the years living as a recluse with an inadequate diet, the elderly woman had become vitamin C deficient and developed scurvy. The anaemia of scurvy is usually normochromic, normocytic and the bruising is of a non-thrombocytopenic, non-blanching-with-pressure variety. The diagnosis was made by serum vitamin C assay and the vitamin C saturation test.

103 E

Dr Dale had the clinical features of atherosclerotic brain damage with lower body Parkinsonism (his face had no PD features). Response to L dopa is poor and transient. A response to donepezil or citalopram would not be expected. Falls in idiopathic parkinsonism are a late feature, but not in the atherosclerotic variety.

104 B

The rate of fall in the eGFR best fits an increasing obstruction to flow of urine at any level, especially bladder and prostrate.

105 D

Unpleasant as the task was it was essential that one had to speak to an administrative/organisational doctor and for him to take on the responsibility of offering help to the sick colleague. To not whistle-blow would have made one complicit with the drug abuse and open to criticism. Gone are the days when the fatuous definition of an alcoholic as 'a person who drank more than his doctor' was considered amusing.

The Defence Societies and the BMA have phone facilities from where expert impartial confidential advice is available. One has to consider patients' safety before that of a fellow registrar needing professional help.

106 A

Ibuprofen has the lowest potential serious gastrointestinal tract toxicity. It is the only 'over-the-counter' NSAID available in Britain, indicating the relatively minor gastric mucosal damage risk. While paracetamol (acetaminophen) is freely available and is strictly classified as a NSAID; it is often thought of as different from 'standard' NSAIDs.

107 C

A home visit may be conducted while the patient is still at home. An OT usually visits homes alone but an accompanying professional colleague is not precluded. An OT's aim is to maximise a patient's ability to perform daily living activities. OTs help patients regain skills of living and provide aids to assist such skills. Sensory aids include a clock with a large dial or the substitution of a flashing light for door or telephone bells.

108 B

Reactivation of old TB foci may occur when a patient is immunocompromised – drugs, alcohol abuse, sub-nourishment. Having had TB does not protect a person from reactivation or reinfection.

109 B

The facial (VII cranial) nerve shares sensory supply to the anterior two thirds of the tongue with the trigeminal (Vth). The posterior third of the tongue receives sensory fibres from the glossopharyngeal (IX) cranial nerve.

110 D

The Barthel index helps quantification of a patient's physical functions irrespective of their aetiology. Repeated incontinence of bowel or bladder scores zero, thereby reducing the maximum score from 20.

111 E

While PD is a disturbance of motor function, there are associated non-motor phenomena – the impulse control disorders (ICD). They include compulsive gambling, hypersexuality, excessive repetitive activity, compulsive buying and excessive aimless wandering. The onset of ICDs tends to follow starting or increasing dopamine therapy. It is postulated that dopamine agonist drugs enhance dopaminergic mechanisms via the mesolimbic system, which is considered to be the brain's reward and reinforcement centre.

112 D

A person retraining their walking abilities may use different frames as their strength and confidence return, starting with two staff members and progressing through a Zimmer frame to a delta rollator. The delta frame has a single multi-directional front wheel and two uni-directional back wheels. It allows continuous walking (a Zimmer induces a stop-start-stop pattern of progression) and good manoeuvrability. A delta walker is often preferred by people with PD.

113 A

The pleural fluid is a transudate (protein concentration < 25 g/L). Of the five possibilities, congestive heart failure is the only cause of a transudate.

114 A

In the hypermetropic (long-sighted) eye, the eyeball is too short (or the cornea too curved), such that light rays focus behind the retina. Hypermetropia is corrected by using a convex lens in front of the cornea. The reverse of the above is true in myopia.

Long-sighted people require reading lenses earlier than others. Additionally, because of their smaller eyes the anterior chamber is narrower, making the person more susceptible to closed-angle glaucoma.

115 B

When a P value is > 0.05 (5%), the result is regarded as statistically insignificant because there was insufficient evidence for a difference to be found. A, C, D and E are correct. Editors tend not to publish papers without statistically significant results.

116 E

The clinical, radiological and laboratory features (low-protein ascitic fluid – back pressure from the right heart leading to a transudate) strongly suggest the diagnosis of constrictive pericarditis. Suggestions A to D are untenable conclusions from the data presented.

117 C

To make an autonomous decision (which may be unwise or unconventional) a person should be able to retain information relevant to the decision, appreciate the information relevant to the decision, appreciate the information in relation to him/herself and be able to weigh the information, balancing risks and benefits so as to make an independent decision.

118 B

The laboratory and x-ray findings are characteristic of 'pseudogout' – 'chondrocalcinosis'. The urate crystals in an acute gouty joint show negative birefringence. Positive birefringence is a feature of calcium pyrophosphate crystals. This arthropathy commonly affects the knee or wrist in elderly people.

119 D

All statements in Question 119 are correct. The most pertinent one for an unrelated male is that the condition is sporadic. Rates of incidence (the number of new cases in a population at a particular time) are of no help in prediction for a specific person.

120 E

Morphia may be used in renal failure. The opioid is suitable for severe pain, causes nausea and vomiting in up to 50% and should be used with a stool softener and an osmotic purge. A dry mouth is an almost invariable consequence of morphia therapy.

121 D

While vigorous exercise is a recognised cause of non-malignant increase in PSA, horse or push-bike riding are not considered to lead to spuriously elevated PSA concentrations. The other four options are well-recognised causes of misleading assay results.

see Hoffman RM. Screening for prostatic cancer. *New England J Med.* 2011; **365**: 2013–19.

122 B

Sarcopenia ('poverty of flesh') is a major feature of frailty and is characterised by progressive loss of muscle mass and reduction in muscle strength and/or impaired physical performance. It adversely affects the ability of an elderly person to remain functionally independent.

see Muscaritoli M *et al.* Consensus definition of sarcopenia. *Clin Nutrit.* 2010; **29**: 154–9.

123 D

Omental cake: this is a description of the CT appearance of omentum when its fat has been replaced by tumour – there is a thick confluent soft tissue mass. The common tumours leading to this appearance are ovary, gastrointestinal, pancreas and breast.

The bamboo spine is the x-ray appearance of long-standing ankylosing spondylitis where the paraspinal ligaments calcify. Looser's zones are pseudofractures and appear as narrow translucent bands at cortical margins of bones. These zones are pathognomic of osteomalacia (adult vitamin D deficiency). A coin lesion is a pulmonary nodule (10–30 mm) of which 50% are malignant and of that 50%, half are adenoma carcinomas. The azygos lobe is a developmental abnormality where the azygos vein loops over a portion of the apical segment of the right upper lung lobe. While there is a characteristic chest x-ray appearance, there are no pathological consequences.

124 D

B-natriuretic peptide (BNP) was raised, reflecting left atrial myocyte stretching as part of the backward pressure of heart failure.

A BNP activity of < 400 pg/ml is normal; the range up to about 800 is inconclusive; a figure > 900 represents heart failure. A dyspnoea of moderate exertion roughly correlates with a BNP between 1500 and 2000. In severe heart failure concentrations in excess of 25 000 are found.

125 A

Mrs Stone had features of a systemic bacterial infection without localising physical signs. The raised alkaline phosphatase pointed to liver or bone; the jaundice and the raised alkaline phosphatase indicated liver disturbance. An ultrasound study showed biliary sludge with gallstones in a dilated (> 9 mm) common bile duct. The presentation of this condition without localising signs is well recognised in the elderly.

126 C

Allopurinol enhances the toxicity of azathioprine. After a few days of full dose allopurinol and azathioprine, fatal bone marrow toxicity may well develop. Azathioprine and allopurinol together are always contraindicated.

The other four choices were acceptable.

127 C

This man with T2DM had an HbA_{1c} figure that was 'too good'. Re-examination of the original diagnostic glucose figures showed that a random glucose concentration of 4.9 was transposed to 9.4 and labelled as a fasting sample. The figure (9.4) is compatible with the diagnosis of T2DM (defined as fasting plasma glucose of ≥ 7.0 mmol/L). In the vignette the albumin-creatinine ratio was in the normal range, again not supporting a diagnosis of diabetes mellitus.

128 C

A sad story but because the tablet horde was mentioned in strict confidence, it could not have been discussed with any third party unless with Mrs Lloyds' express permission. Choices A and B would have been reasonable actions.

129 E

Worldwide, dehydration is the commonest explanation. Within hospital practice undesirable consumption of unnecessary or excessive doses of hypotensive drugs is frequently found, as are the consequences of hypovolumemic-inducing diuretics. Diabetes mellitus is the commonest cause of autonomic failure hypotension.

Often an explanation for postural hypotension is not found.

130 E

Descending from A to E is increasing strength and thus better quality levels of evidence. A meta-analysis combines the results of several studies and gives a single confidence interval for a given intervention. Additionally a large-scale, multi-centre, well-designed randomised controlled trial (D) provides very strong evidence of controlled activities.

131 D

If a COPD patient is in a stable lung state some weeks after the last exacerbation and the PaO_2 is < 7.3 whilst breathing air (SaO_2 on air ≤ 88%) on two separate occasions at least 3 weeks apart, then long-term oxygen therapy (LTOT) will be of help. The possibilities A, B, C and E are not indications for LTOT because no benefit has been demonstrated.

There is little evidence that short-burst oxygen therapy gives any benefit to COPD patients other than that of a psychological nature.

132 D

Bradykinesia is one of the four principal features of Parkinson's disease; the others are rigidity, flexed posture and tremor. Features A, B, C and E either favour the diagnosis of essential tremor or carry no differential diagnostic weight.

133 C

Bladder catheter urine will always contain some protein and leucocytes as a consequence of catheter trauma to urethra and bladder mucosa. Bacteria are always grown from a CSU. Urinary catheters have local pressure effects – tissue necrosis, haematuria and the introduction of bacteria. Bacteria grown from CSU samples are not necessarily pathogens or responsible for symptoms.

134 C

Hammer toes show hyperextension at the metatarsophalangeal joints and fixed flexion at interphalangeal joints. The other statements are correct.

135 B

The clinical features and presence of HLA B27 all support the diagnosis. This is typically painful and progressive. An x-ray showed calcification of the inter-vertebral ligaments with disc ossification and squaring of vertebral bodies. The sacro-spinal ligaments were lost by bony ankylosis. These are the typical radiological features of ankylosing spondylitis.

136 C

This academic had full mental capacity and was aware of the consequences of his decision. His wishes were respected because a competent person may make choices which lead to their discomfort, danger or death regardless of other people's opinions.

137 B

The declarative episodic memory is the ability to recall recent facts and events. It depends on the hippocampus and associated structures in the medial temporal lobe. The semantic memory involves vocabulary and recall of events in the long past; working memory includes mental arithmetic and abstract reasoning; the procedural, involves complex trained motor skills.

138 A

A simple drug regime is always best. Choice A is straightforward and is an appropriate dose for a small elderly woman with adequate renal function. Suggestions B and C require what may be unrealistic complexity. Dose D was too high for age and eGFR. Option E expected the elderly patient to snap a tablet and save half-tablet doses day to day: neither sensible nor practicable.

139 C

Auramine phenol staining is used as a screening procedure for alcohol-acid-fast bacilli (AAFB) detection. If present ZN stains are used for confirmation. The finding of AAFB on a ZN-stained sputum smear virtually establishes the diagnosis. If AAFB are not seen at microscopy, they may be recovered by LJ culture. Should clinical matters be urgent an assay for circulating interferon γ (IFNγ) is appropriate. The test system detects IFNγ released by T-lymphocytes which have responded to MTB specific antigens. A positive IFNγ test is tantamount to diagnosing re-activation of MTB infection.

140 C

Depression was the principal diagnosis and was treated with an antidepressant. The geriatric depression score was 7/15, which equates to 'moderate depression'.

see Lester H, Gilbody S. Choosing a second generation antidepressant for treatment of MDD. *BMJ*. 2012; **344**: 11.

141 B

Mrs Ample had severe obesity (class II; BMI 35–39.9). Her data showed the co-existence of major risk factors for cardiovascular events – hypertension, hyperglycaemia and hypertriglycaemia fulfilling the criteria for metabolic syndrome. Additionally there was insulin resistance – acanthosis nigricans and T2DM.

Related to deranged metabolic factors there was a non-alcoholic steatohepatitis (fatty liver, raised γGT and ALT), ECG evidence of ischaemic heart disease and an early diabetic nephropathy as shown by the detection of microalbuminuria.

Mrs Ample had a reduced quality of life and a shortened life expectation.

see Bailey CJ. The challenge of managing coexistent T2DM and obesity. *BMJ*. 2011; **342**: 913–18.

142 A

About 2 million people die of malaria per annum and very largely are members of third-world countries which for many additional reasons have a life expectancy substantially less than first-world populations.

The 'grey' currency is the free disposable income of the retired. Such people enjoy affluence which positively correlates with enhanced longevity and political influence.

see Mulley G. Myths of ageing. *Clin Med.* 2007; **7**: 68–72.

143 D

Serum PTH values increase with age, which correlates with a fall in vitamin D activity. The combined effect presumably contributes to age-related reduction in bone mass – osteomalacia. A, B and E are correct.

144 C

A, B, D and E are correct. Arcus corneae have no pathological association. Shortening of the axial length of the eyeball is the normal anatomical change occurring with increasing age. Hypermetropia (presbyopia) is the consequence of the axial reduction. (see also Answer 114)

145 A

It has been clearly documented that obsessional attention to oral hygiene reduces the number of aspiration episodes. The other listed conditions are likely to increase the risk of food or fluid inhalation.

146 E

The padded shell of the hip protector lies over the greater trochanter and softens the trauma of a fall but not the frequency. Items A to D all increase the risk of a fall. About a third of people over 65 years old fall each year.

see de Rooikj SE. Hip protectors to prevent femoral fractures. *BMJ.* 2006; **332**: 559. Close JCT, Lord SR. Falls assessment in older people. *BMJ.* 2011; **343**: 579–82.

147 A

While all five possible actions might have been appropriate, a sexual history should have been taken first. The patient may not have indulged in any sexual activity, legitimate or otherwise.

148 E

Pethidine is a short-acting opioid not appropriate for chronic pain management. Oxycodone is useful and up to × 1.5 stronger than morphine. Methadone has a different receptor-binding pattern from the μ opioid agonists. It can provide superior analgesia to morphia and has a better side-effect profile. Fentanyl is delivered transcutaneously and the 'patch' has to be replaced every 72 hours. It is used in conjunction with morphine. Buprenorphine also has transdermal delivery; the 'patch' is changed weekly. Transdermal delivery of both fentanyl and buprenorphine take 24 to 72 hours before steady plasma concentrations are gained from starting or increasing the dose. A fentanyl '12' patch is the approximate equivalent of 45 mg morphine sulphate if applied for 24 hours in a steady state across a healthy skin.

149 C

The MCV was low, which suggested a microcytic anaemia. With all probability the anaemia was iatrogenic – an aspirin-induced gastritis. The blood urea was disproportionately raised to the normal creatinine concentration – suggesting a sudden gut bleed from the gastric mucosa with digestion of the erythrocytes on a background of chronic iron deficiency (MCV 76).

150 B

Wynn Jones had a typical history of allergic bronchopulmonary aspergillosis. The allergic component was shown by the eosinophilia, the raised total IgE and the considerably raised IgE RAST (radio allergosorbent test) at > 100 000 KU/L. A RAST measures an allergen specific IgE – in this case, antibodies against *Aspergillus fumigatus*. This result secured the diagnosis.

151 B

The question described a patient with an insidious onset of temporal arteritis (giant cell arteritis) and separated it from other suggested conditions.

152 A

In clinical practice a number of variables would have been assayed simultaneously but the first discriminating test was to find that a random plasma glucose figure was 13.9 – more than 11.1 – the cut off between glucose intolerance and T2DM.

153 A

The low plasma sodium and urinary abnormalities are characteristic features of Legionnaire's disease. They do not 'fit' the other listed conditions. Urinalysis is usually within normal limits in patients with lung conditions with the exception of *L. pneumophila* infection.

154 A

Either a β-blocker or calcium channel blockers (CCB) are first choice drugs. Atenolol and bisoprolol are relatively cardioselective and are widely used. With care, they may be used in COPD (see Answer 323). Of the CCBs, verapamil is often used but the negative inotropic property can precipitate heart failure. Verapamil should not be combined with any β-blocker because of the risk of hypotension and asystole. Nifepidine or amlodipine are effective in angina and easier to use.

see Krause T *et al.* Management of hypertension: summary of NICE guidelines. *BMJ*. 2011; **343**: 418–20.

155 E
All five factors increase the risk of a stroke, but hypertension is the strongest.

156 A
About 70% of all leg ulcers are venous – thus the majority of leg ulcers develop over the course of the long saphenous vein. Ideally an ulcerated leg should be elevated above heart level but in many elderly people this is not feasible. Lipodermatosclerosis (thickening of dermis and subcutis) is a measure of chronic venous ulceration. Deep 'punched out' ulcers are arterial. The APBI is 1 to 1.2 in persons with an adequate leg arterial supply. The application of pressure bandaging to a leg with an APBI < 0.8 risks iatrogenic gangrene.

157 D
Apathy is a feature of the 'Parkinson plus' condition, progressive supranuclear palsy, not PD itself.

158 C
Elderly people with biventricular failure may never have the classical symptoms of dyspnoea, orthopnea, paroxysmal nocturnal dyspnoea and ankle swelling. Lethargy and fatigue often reflect a wide range of different disease processes. Low-dose furosemide and perindopril set her on her way.

159 C
This man had developed a nephrotic syndrome – peripheral pitting oedema (weight gain), hypoalbuminaemia and 'heavy' proteinuria (urine protein: creatinine ratio > 350 mg/mmol or > 4.5 g/ 24 hours). Protein solutions froth when stirred – urine in the lavatory pan. Nephrotic syndrome results from a glomerular leak of serum protein in excess of tubular reabsorptive capacity and hepatic synthetic rates. No particular range of GFR is associated with the nephrotic state (CKD 3Ap – eGFR 45–59 ml/min/1.73 m², 'p' indicating substantial proteinuria). The GFR in a nephrotic person can range from 100% to zero – a few patients remain nephrotic on dialysis.

Congestive cardiac failure is not associated with hypoalbuminaemia and 'heavy' proteinuria. While albumin synthesis is reduced in advanced liver disease, proteinuria is not a feature.

160 B
Within approximately 10 years, about 50% of individuals who sustain a meniscal injury develop osteoarthritis. The synovial fluid data fit this diagnosis. In farmers there is an association between OA of the hip and their occupation, but not of the knee.

161 D

There is nothing in the vignette to support A or E. Wilson's disease rarely presents later than middle age; the majority of cases are diagnosed in childhood and adolescence. Primary biliary cirrhosis is classically a disease of middle-aged women. There is a well-recognised association between night sweats and lymphoma. This malignancy was diagnosed via liver biopsy.

162 E

This appears intuitive but:

1 repair and maintenance is not excessively costly to the organism
2 day-to-day nutritional cost is high – in nature many die of starvation
3 the DST suggests that post-menopausal women would not age
4 females use more resources in reproduction, therefore men should live longer than they do
5 a limited lifespan should be species advantageous by allowing more food to be available for organisms during their reproductive period

Essentially the DST explains ageing by asking how best an organism should allocate its metabolic resources – for day-to-day survival and the production of progeny. The DST has attracted much interest and currently is the chief theoretical explanation of ageing in sexually reproducing species.

see Kirkwood TBL, Austad SN. Why do we age? *Nature*. 2000; **408**: 233–8.

163 B

Fifty patients would need to receive and take hypotensive drugs to prevent one further brain attack. The relative risk reduction (95% confidence interval) being approximately 30% (15–40). Blood pressure reduction is the single most important intervention in secondary stroke prevention. Answer A data referred to the NNT as a primary prevention strategy.

If the stroke risk is 2% per annum and treatment prevents 50% of strokes (relative risk 50%), treating 100 patients for 1 year will prevent one stroke; NNT 100. The higher the risk, the smaller the NNT for effective therapy.

164 B

The signs described are diagnostic of a III cranial (oculomotor) nerve paralysis including parasympathetic fibres. Ptosis – paralysis of levator palpebrae superioris. Fixed dilated pupil – parasympathetic. The deviation out of the eye is due to the unopposed action of the superior oblique muscle (IV, trochlea) and the downward gaze consequent upon the unopposed medial rectus (VI, abducens).

An acute, isolated, painful, unilateral III palsy is very commonly due to compression by an unruptured aneurysm of the posterior communicating artery.

165 E

The 'full' face symptom and physical signs are characteristic of the condition. Metastatic lung cancer is easily the commonest cause. Sid Perks required urgent admission to hospital, 16 mg dexamethasone daily and an endocaval stent whilst dealing with the malignancy.

166 D

The pearly umbilicated nodules of molluscum contagiosum are common in children and young adults, not the elderly.

167 D

This syndrome comprises unpleasant feelings in the legs which worsen when drowsy but improve with movement or treatment (see Answer 6). The other four choices are well-recognised causes of hypersomnolence.

168 A

There is no established route for elder abuse management (previously called 'granny battering'). Social services, caring agencies, local health officials, the general practitioner and perhaps the police need to be consulted.

169 C

The IGT definition requires the fasting plasma glucose to be < 7.0 and the 2-hour OGGT ≥ 7.8 and 11.0. If the plasma glucose is ≥ 11.1 (as in C) the patient has diabetes mellitus.

see Farmer A, Fox R. Diagnosis, classification and treatment of diabetes mellitus. *BMJ*.2011; **343**: 597–8.

170 D

An important feature of the practice of geriatric medicine is always, if possible, to trim the (often) excessive number of drugs prescribed and swallowed by compliant elderly people. It is quick and easy to prescribe while thought and discontinuation of drugs takes time. The definition of polypharmacy is too restrictive for patients, for example, with heart failure but reflects a sound general principle. In good clinical geriatric practice one should aim to withdraw more drugs than prescribe. Rewarding a surgery visit or hospital appointment with an FP10 is traditional but not necessarily desirable.

Primum non nocere.

171 D

The vagus (X). This cranial is also involved with phonation and also supplies sensory and motor fibres to the oesophagus.

172 A

In young people, *Neisseria gonorrhoeae* is the most common cause of a septic arthritis but in a septuagenarian, *Staphylococcus aureus* is much more likely to be cultured. *Haemophilus influenzae* causes septic arthritis in children; *Strep viridians*, subacute bacterial endocarditis; and *N meningitides*, meningococcal septicaemia.

173 A

Fred had developed a dehydration stone, found in people who live in very warm climates and have an inadequate fluid intake, leading to the production of small volumes of highly concentrated urine. The metabolic screen, as expected, was negative. Metabolic renal stones develop in younger people. Ultrasound studies of the renal tract are insensitive to stones. Of the possibilities A to E, only A and B are diagnosable at cystoscopy; a transitional cell carcinoma does not cause perineal pain and dysuria.

174 D

An acute attack of gout should be treated without stopping urate-lowering drugs; colchicine was the correct treatment for Mr Fry. An increase in allopurinol would not provide relief; it might worsen matters. It should have been continued in unchanged dose. An NSAID is contraindicated on account of the renal failure.

see Ellis S, Koduri G. Crystal Arthropies. *Medicine.* 2010; **38**: 146–50.
Neog T. Gout. *New Engl J Med.* 2011; **364**: 443–52.

175 C

Prof Cor had the symptoms and signs of advanced aortic stenosis; untreated, his life expectancy would have been 2 years or less. The stenotic valve constituted a mechanical, not medical, matter: valve replacement either via an open heart approach or via a stent-mounted valve introduced via the femoral artery is needed promptly (TAVI: transcatheter aortic valve implantation). The choice of drugs in D were inappropriate because they would have reduced the pre-load, thereby worsening the already compromised left ventricular ejection fraction. Likewise the drugs suggested in option E show an inadequate understanding of the pathophysiology and urgency of the case.

176 D

From the description given, hyponatraemia is the only abnormal finding. The selective serotonin reuptake inhibitor, venlafaxine is the most likely drug to have induced inappropriate antidiuretic hormone secretion and hence a plasma sodium of 122. Venlafaxine may also induce constipation and impair memory.

see Wakil A, Ng JM, Atkins S. Investigation of hyponatraemia. *BMJ.* 2011; **342**: 594–6.

177 E

Hypophosphataemia is a feature of the refeeding syndrome which develops if a malnourished patient is supplied feed at too high a rate. Cells rapidly take up phosphate, magnesium and potassium such that the serum concentrations of these electrolytes become subnormal. A less concentrated enteral feed, which can gradually be increased to full strength over weeks, is required.

see Ziegler TR. Nutritional support in critical illness. *New Engl J Med.* 2011; **365**: 562–64.

178 E

A Gleason score of 6 indicates a well-differentiated tumour. The PSA of 13 ng/ml was only very modestly raised and there was no evidence of metastatic spread. Those factors together with 'TC's' age of 84 years indicated that no active treatment was needed. The PSA was measured at six-monthly intervals. Treatment might have been indicated if the PSA had risen – implying spread to bones, but 'TC' finally died of bronchopneumonia aged 89, at which stage there was no evidence of metastatic spread.

see Hoffman RM. Screening for prostatic cancer. *New Engl J Med.* 2011; **365**: 2013–19. Swallow T, Chowdhury S, Kirby RS. Cancer of the prostate gland. *Medicine.* 2012; **40**: 10–13.

179 A

Repeated visits to a doctor at frequent intervals with the same symptoms and with the inability to accept reassurance is hypochondriacal behaviour. Hypochondriacal personalities have *idées fixes* regarding contracting or having a serious disease. They cannot be persuaded to the contrary. There is an unrealistic interpretation of physical sensations and symptoms, which persists despite medical evaluation, investigation and reassurance.

180 E

The diagnosis was very likely to be *Clostridium difficile* (CD) infection from the timing of onset of symptoms and the fact that the patient had been treated with an inappropriate antibiotic. For a straightforward urinary tract infection, trimethoprim or nitrofurantoin are the drugs of first choice.

When CD toxin is detected from a fresh case, treatment comprises vancomycin or metronidazole orally for 10–14 days. Success of treatment is judged by cessation of diarrhoea. Repeat assay for CD toxin is not needed because the toxin may continue to be excreted for months in an asymptomatic person.

see Settle C, Kerr KG. Diarrhoea after broad spectrum antibiotics. *BMJ.* 2011; **243**: 152–3.

181 A

The CAGE questions are:
    B Cut down
    C Annoyed
    D Guilt
    E Eye opener

The CAGE screening tool for alcohol abuse is widely used: a single positive answer to any of the four questions is suggestive of an alcohol problem. If two replies are positive, the sensitivity and specificity of there being an alcohol problem are approximately 90%.

see Holmwood C. Alcohol and drug problems in other people. *BMJ*. 2012; **344**: 7–8.

182 B
Urine sodium excretion was disproportionate to the plasma sodium concentration. Physiologically, urine sodium excretion should cut back to correct the hyponatraemia. The urine sodium concentration was inappropriately high to plasma osmolality. Likewise and reflecting the sodium abnormalities, urinary osmolality was inappropriately high to plasma osmolality. The figures in Question 182 are typical of Syndrome of Inappropriate Anti-Diuretic Hormone (SIADH).

183 A
While relatives have the right to information about DNAR orders, with the consent of a competent patient, they do not have the right to insist on alteration of a senior medical decision about resuscitation status.

184 E
The neuroleptic malignant syndrome is a complication of the use of neuroleptic drugs (haloperidol, chlorpromazine, risperidone) in which there is fever, rigidity and tremor. A to D are all recognised possible consequences of antidepressant drugs.

185 D
The son is not ill but requires help while his elderly mother recovers. An acute hospital bed is not the correct placement for the son; a period of respite care would have been appropriate. If D was not possible, A would have been a solution.

186 D
The majority of men with diabetes over the age of 50 years have erectile dysfunction (ED) and the incidence increases with the passage of years. The prevalence of ED in non-diabetic septuagenarians is about 20–25% in Britain.

187 D
Whilst lying on her kitchen floor, there was prolonged pressure on Mrs Prescott's skeletal muscles causing necrosis and release of myoglobin. The muscle protein precipitates in renal tubules, causing obstruction to the flow of urine. The acute renal failure (acute kidney injury) following rhabdomyolysis is one of the pigment nephropathies. Raised concentrations of myoglobin in blood or urine are diagnostic.

188 B

The first consideration was the resident's safety in her new surroundings. Thus, advice and perhaps aids for living from an occupational therapist could well be beneficial before other matters were addressed. Financial benefits are available for the registered blind.

see Cupples ME *et al.* Improving healthcare access for people with visual impairment. *BMJ.* 2012; **343**: 42–9.

189 E

Mirtazapine is an SNRI and is an alternative to an SSRI such as citalopram or fluoxetine. An advantage of mirtazapine is that it has a sedative component which is of benefit in poor sleepers. Switching from an SSRI to an SNRI was appropriate strategy. Changing to a Monoamine oxidase inhibitor (MAOI) is a specialist decision.

190 A

Ms Tripp's footwear may have been worn and dangerous. She might have fallen in a particular part of her home, suggesting a local hazard such as a loose rug or a linoleum defect. Postural hypotension had to be excluded. TFT: hypothyroidism causes muscular weakness and hyperthyroidism arrhythmias. Insufficient detail was supplied to suggest an x-ray investigation.

see Close J, Lord S. Fall assessment in older people. *BMJ.* 2011; **343**: 579–82.

191 E

Achalasia was the most likely diagnosis. The 18-month history made a carcinoma unlikely. The diagnosis of achalasia was made at upper gastrointestinal endoscopy and clinched by oesophageal manometric observations. Achalasia is a condition of the middle-aged and older.

192 D

Joan Hunter Dunn would have needed a few weeks to acclimatise fully to her new life before she was realistically able to consider her advanced care plans. By then she had had the time to gain confidence in her new environment and with the care home staff.

193 B

The aide-memoire involving the 'I's' comprises the following: intellectual failure, incontinence, immobility, instability and iatrogenic illness.

see Evans JG. Geriatrics. *Clin Med.* 2011; **11**: 166–8.

194 A

A teaspoon is preferred to a tablespoon – the volume of food delivered from a loaded tablespoon may well be too large, impairing food bolus movement in the mouth and potentially 'flooding' the swallowing mechanisms. If music is played, it should be harmonious and tranquil, not discordant, displeasing and disagreeable, with the volume adjusted to the feedee's comfortable hearing. Classical FM at low volume is ideal (FM 100–102 MHz).

195 A

The description of the blistering disorder in Question 195 is typical of bullous pemphigoid. There a similarities to pemphigus but the latter develops in younger people and requires more potent therapy.

196 C

Diamorphine can be mixed with any of the following, singly or together: cyclizine, dextramethasone, haloperidol, hyoscine, metoclopramide or midazolam and infused subcutaneously. Suggestions A to D are valid.

197 C

The dull percussion note excludes a pneumothorax and suggests an effusion or parenchymal consolidation. Tactile vocal fremitus is reduced in the presence of an effusion but may be increased in association with consolidation.

198 B

There is increased sympathetic tone during exercise which increases myocardial rate and contractions. Digoxin enhances muscular contractions and slows the heart by increasing vagal tone. The sympathetic drive of exercise overrides the vagal/digoxin slowing with loss of drug efficiency. Thus the active person in whom atrial fibrillation has to be controlled should be treated not with digoxin alone but with bisoprolol or a calcium channel blocker such as diltiazem alone or in combination with digoxin.

199 E

Such a patient has very limited thoracic reserve due to respiratory muscle weakness. Coughing would be weak and the individual persistently at risk of aspiration. Intra-abdominal instrumentation would further reduce life expectation.

200 B

Muehrke, an American renal physician, described white transverse bands on the nails occurring in severe hypoalbuminaemia. There is no association with malignancy.

201 D

While it is likely that the generator pouch was infected, attempts at aspiration could have damaged the leads. An echo might have shown tricuspid vegetations where a lead passed through the valve. Antibiotics were not used until blood culture results were available.

202 C

The MRI features are those of TB infection (Pott's disease) and of cord compression causing upper motor neurone features with spastic weakness and sensory loss. The painless progression of the condition is typical of a cold abscess in an elderly person.

Mycobacterium tuberculosis organisms invade vertebral bodies without involvement of the disks – an osteomyelitis. Subsequently the infection then spreads to adjacent vertebral disks – diskitis. Conversely, with other bacterial infections the vertebral body end plates are involved. The most common infectious organisms are Staphylococcal and Enterobacter species.

203 D

While many old people have to spend > 10% of their income on heating, 'fuel-poor households' are not confined to the elderly. The topic became politically important during the 2011/12 winter which followed the stonking August 2011 increases in gas and electricity prices in Britain.

204 B

The woman was severely B_{12} deficient (52 ng/L; 150–1000). The peripheral neuropathy and mental changes were a consequence of the deficiency. Pancytopenia is a feature of this state and jaundice results from premature red cell destruction in the circulation and marrow.

Replacement therapy corrected the haematology and biochemistry, and helped the cerebral dysfunction but the neuropathy persisted.

205 B

Infection with *Neisseria gonorrhoeae* was the most likely explanation of dysuria and abundant discharge. Chlamydia infection is usually asymptomatic but may produce similar symptoms but with a less obvious discharge. A discharge is not a feature of a 'standard' urinary tract infection or a non-specific urethritis. Genital herpes is associated with systemic symptoms followed by a painful vesicular genital rash.

Because this man was in his seventies it did not follow that he was not sexually active.

206 E

While Mr Sugar needed 'sorting out' there was an urgent priority to save his declining vision by laser photocoagulation. Given his disinterest in his health, it would have been unlikely that he would have benefited from insulin. Before consulting a kidney doctor, a renal ultrasound was needed to investigate the possibility of an additional component to his (presumed) nephropathy.

207 B

Section 7 concerns guardianship. In the Question 207 scenario, a guardian would be appointed rapidly and have the authority to require access to be given for doctors and social workers where the individual lived. The guardian also would have the authority to insist on attendance at a hospital or surgery for treatment.

Rose Flower's case might have been considered under Section 47 of the National Assistance Act 1948. This Act allows the removal of an individual held to be at severe risk at home, but who refuses to go to hospital.

208 C

Both C and D are correct but because so many middle-aged patients are expected to take PPIs for their final 30 years, hypochlorhydria is common. Many, if not the majority of indications for long-term PPIs chiefly benefit the manufacturer's profits more than those who are burdened with their consumption.

209 D

The Barthel index is an assessment of daily activities and their restrictions that people actually achieve in their daily lives including the use of aids and devices. See Answer 311 concerning aids and devices.

210 A

This is a clear-cut case where a patient with Parkinson's disease was treated with a dopamine receptor antagonist (haloperidol) inducing an orofacial tardive dyskinesia. Over a period of years it may remit after cessation of the haloperidol or other neuroleptic drug.

see Mackin P, Thomas SHL. Atypical anti-psychotic drugs. *BMJ*. 2011; **342**: 650–4.

211 A

The first step (NICE 2011) is to establish whether the patient has an elevated BP. A single figure recorded at what was probably a stressful time is of limited value. Repeating the pressure measurement by the practitioner after the Surgery Sister has done so is unlikely to gain a reliable baseline pressure. Clinically, there was no urgency and a 24-hour ambulatory BP monitor is a much more accurate, cost-effective way of deciding whether the patient had or had not sustained elevation of his blood pressure. Too many people of all ages are prescribed hypotensive drugs without their doctors taking the trouble to establish a diagnosis. A geriatrician is likely to stop far more potentially or actually harmful hypotensive medications rather than prescribe such drugs. In many cases it is likely that the manufacturer's profits benefit more than those swallowing pills for years.

NICE suggests that a patient with a sustained BP > 140/90 should be offered pressure-lowering treatment. In elderly people, the prescriber should have a clear therapeutic aim in mind before pressing drugs upon asymptomatic and possibly frail people.

Primum non nocere

see Richie LD, Campbell NC, Murchie P. New NICE guidelines for hypertension. *BMJ*. 2011; **343**: 491–2.

212 E

A full upper and lower set of dentures is more frequently found in people from reduced social backgrounds. The frequency at which dentures are required is diminishing. This will improve the quality of life of those who are able to retain their teeth and also help with maintenance of oral hygiene. Dentures – fitted oral plastic prostheses – are not preferred at any age, although many elderly people think of their acquisition as a normal part of ageing. Toothache is abolished and the difficulty of finding and paying for dental care is over.

213 C

During a full discussion it was explained to the relatives that the MDT's opinion could, reluctantly, be strengthened by a court direction. The well-meaning relatives then appreciated the value of professional views and agreed to arrange the home for the receipt of Mrs Law's equipment and substantial support package. It was not fair or realistic for an elderly husband and granddaughter to supply around-the-clock help for an elderly woman needing much assistance (Barthel 10/20). The relatives would have failed adequately to cope and Mrs Law would have required a further hospital admission.

see The NHS & Community Care Act 1990

214 D

The clues to the diagnosis were the stiff collar, the 'faint' following a particular neck movement and the post-prandial timing. The upward-angled, stiff-collared neck pressed on Sir Perry's carotid sinus, leading to a sinus pause of 4–5 seconds which he interpreted as a 'faint'. The diagnosis was made in a vascular laboratory where carotid sinus massage (a test for carotid sinus hypersensitivity) reproduced the 'faint'. Later that day Sir Perry had a dual-chamber pacemaker inserted in the Portland Hospital.

Carotid sinus syndrome is an abnormal haemodynamic response to carotid sinus stimulation. It induces a strong bradycardic reflex resulting in sinus pauses, at times with complete heart block.

215 C

Renal tract TB was established from culture of Early Morning Urine (EMU) samples. Investigation showed that ureteric oedema had led to a left autonephrectomy and severe obstructive damage to the right kidney. An offer of dialysis was declined.

About 70% of new cases of TB in the UK are diagnosed in people who were born overseas. In almost half, the site of infection is extrapulmonary. The highest rates of TB are found in sub-Saharan Africa but TB is very prominent in densely populated areas of China and India.

see Friedland JS. Tuberculosis in the 21st century. *Clin Med.* 2011; **11**: 353–7.

Sheerin NS. Urinary tract infection. *Medicine.* 2011; **39**: 384–9.

216 D

An orthosis is a device worn outside the body which supports and helps the function of that part to which it is applied. By that definition, a denture is not an orthosis, while a cosmetic nose replacement is. Dentures are prostheses.

217 C

Visual disturbance is a well-known symptom of excessive digoxin doses. In some people, yellow-green tinged vision (xanthopsia) is a consequence. Investigations showed Mr Withering's blood concentration of digoxin to be 4.5 ng/ml (therapeutic range 0.9–2.0). He had been prescribed digoxin at too high a dose for his renal excretory capabilities (eGFR 28).

The original William Withering was a GP in Birmingham who first identified the diuretic benefit of a foxglove infusion in some patients with 'dropsy'. He published his observations in 1785.

218 C

Miss Spy had developed bilateral cataracts (opacification of the crystalline lens) and she was listed for surgical treatment. Cataracts in their earlier stages characteristically lead to impaired vision in low light. Briefly:

> chronic glaucoma – affects perhaps 5% of people > 70 years old. As it progresses there is peripheral followed by central field loss.

> diabetic retinopathy – may be diagnosed in the early years of T2DM; the hallmark is a proliferative retinopathy in which new blood vessels grow forward into the vitreous humour.

> retinitis pigmentosa – causes gradual loss of peripheral fields leading to tunnel vision. The worst varieties of RP lead to a visual acuity of < 6/60 by 50 years – this corresponds to being partially sighted.

> ARMD – leads to loss of central vision. The wet variety has a successful treatment available (A20).

see Chakravarthy U, Evans J, Rosenfeld PJ. Age related macular degeneration. *BMJ.* 2010; **340**: 526–30.

219 D

This man began work in a dockyard decades before mesothelioma was recognised as asbestos related and before health and safety regulations had been formulated. Blue asbestos was widely used as an insulating agent without protection of the workers from airborne fibres.

The plaques (shown on CXR) relate to blue fibre exposure but are not pre-malignant. Clubbing may occur in both mesothelioma and lung cancer; in this case its presence was non-discriminatory.

220 A

Onchocerciasis (river blindness) is a filarial infection caused by *Onchocerca volvulus*, which is an important cause of cataract in tropical Africa. Onycholysis is the painless loosening of a nail from its bed; onychogryphosis (ram's horn) is the deformity of thickened, untrimmed nails; onychomycosis is fungal nail infection and onychocryptosis occurs where inadequately trimmed nails damage the nail sulcus, allowing infection to develop.

221 C

The five Fried's indicators of frailty are weight loss, exhaustion, low energy expenditure, weakness and slowness. An elderly person with none of these is considered to be robust. Three or more indicators constitute frailty.

see Hubbard RE, O'Mahony S, Woodhouse KW. Characterising frailty in the elderly setting. *Age & Ageing.* 2009; **38**: 115–19.

222 C

The β-lactamase-stable β-lactam (co-amoxiclav) covers *Streptococcus pneumoniae* (the commonest cause of CAP) and the macrolide (clarithromycin) covers 'atypical' causes of pneumonia – *Mycoplasma pneumoniae*, *Legionella pneumophila*, Q fever and psittacosis.

223 E

The choice of B seems obvious but Mr Ali and other devout Muslims are prepared to set aside physical hazard. Some elderly Muslims hope to die in Mecca, thereby perhaps gaining an extra blessing. Infirmity is therefore not a major consideration for pious adherents of Islam when undertaking their essential pilgrimage.

see Gatrad AR, Sheikh A. The Hajj. *BMJ.* 2011; **343**: 637–8.

224 C

Thoracolumbar and mid-thoracic levels are the most common sites at which osteoporotic fractures occur. Conversely, fracture-related disability tends to be greater in patients with lumbar fractures than among those with thoracic fractures.

225 A

The JVP was raised by 7 cm and there were persistent crepitations at both bases. Furosemide was prescribed and in 14 days Mrs Woodland had lost 3.5 kg. The BNP pre-treatment was 6100 ng/L (reference range < 400). With diuretic control of the expanded circulating volume the back pressure on liver and kidneys returned to normal, as shown by cessation of the hyperbilirubinaemia, return of the eGFR to previous values and fall of BNP to below 400.

226 E

Flattened small bowel villi are a hallmark of coeliac disease, the diagnosis of which is supported by the demonstration of antibodies against tissue transglutaminase (tTG). A gluten-free diet reverses the histological and laboratory features and improves overall health and longevity.

227 D

One of the early features of PD is reduced arm swing. There may be no tremor at presentation. In Mr Black's case levodopa allowed the arm to swing normally, thereby winding the watch, and it also reversed other PD features.

228 E

If fewer children are born, the ratio young:elderly alters in the direction of the older population.

see Myint PK, Welch AA. Healthier aging. *BMJ*. 2012; **344**: 42–5.

229 E

The capillary glucose figures pre-breakfast and supper stand out as needing attention. Better 24-hour control should be possible by using the long-acting insulin glargine (> 24-hour activity) and judging a pre-meal dose of a short-acting (about 2 hours) insulin such as lispro or aspart. Because Mrs Sphere was a sporty type, the greater flexibility in glucose control gained by lispro use was an additional advantage.

230 A

The AA is claimed by an individual for the benefit of their carer. The following criteria have to be fulfilled:
1   the claimant has to be > 65 years old
2   there has to be an expectation that the disability will last > 6 months
3   the claimant is resident in quarters not state or council funded.

Help for night care may be claimable. If a person is expected to die within 3 months, extra cash (via 'fast track') may be available. Information to guide patient or carer through the maze may be found via a Citizen's Advice Bureau or the charity Age UK (see the Yellow Pages or their websites).

231 E

If a patient without mental capacity is abandoned in an NHS ward, a mechanism exists for a senior hospital officer to act in the best interests of the abandoned and authorise transfer to a suitable institution.

232 C

The physical signs are those of a spastic paraplegia. Localisation is provided because the umbilical region is supplied by neurones from D10. As a rough guide the following dermatomes innervate at the following levels:

C4   shoulders
T4   nipples
T10 umbilicus
L1   iliac crest
L3   knee
S1   lateral feet

233 C

Extramammary Paget's disease presents with persistent red plaques in the anogenital region or auxiliary sites. There is no breast component of the condition.

234 C

The WHO pain relief ladder applies:

non-opioid – paracetamol, NSAIDs
weak opioid – codeine, tramadol
strong opioid – morphine, fentanyl

The correct step was to combine paracetamol with codeine phosphate, thereby keeping the strong opioid for later use.

235 A

Constipation in PD is extremely common from the early stages of the disease. In some, overflow occurs. Faecal incontinence is also found in multiple system atrophy syndrome – one of the Parkinson plus syndromes. Before ascribing faecal leaking to the PD colon, colorectal cancer has to be excluded.

236 E

Calcification of cartilage is an important feature in establishing the diagnosis of pyrophosphate arthropathy.

237 E

Competence is decision specific. It needs to be assessed for a particular question/decision or planned important decision. Previously established competency does not allow one to assume that it still holds when new significant matters need decisions.

238 C

The 2011 NICE updated recommendations concerning management of hypertension suggest that patients aged 80+ years should be treated as for similar people aged 60–80. The overall health of octogenarians varies considerably, thus selection of patients is essential. Treatment of all is incorrect. Many elderly people suffer from injudicious and often unnecessary hypotensive medication. Target blood pressure figures must be realistic and achieved without patient harm. In hospital practice it is often necessary to stop hypotensive drugs which once perhaps were required but the indication having long been superseded. The continued ingestion of unnecessary chemicals risks the patient's health and is wasteful.

Primum non nocere

see Mancia G. Antihypertensives in octogenarians. *BMJ*. 2012; **343**: 8.

239 C

The TSH assay should be repeated in 2–3 months because often an isolated, mildly raised TSH activity spontaneously reverts to normal.

240 D

In primary open-angle glaucoma with advancing vision loss, peripheral visual fields are lost first. Untreated, tunnel vision develops, followed by blindness.

241 E

In a kidney supplied via stenosed renal artery, glomerular perfusion is dependent upon intra-renal angiotensin II maintenance of glomerular filtration. An ACEI blocks A II production, leading to prompt deterioration in kidney filtration. Arteriosclerotic, rather than fibromuscular dysplasia renal artery stenosis is the likely morphology in an older person.

242 B

Timolol may be absorbed systemically after topical application to the eye. Bradycardia leading to heart block is a well-recognised consequence – as in the vignette. While urine infections in elderly people often cause confusion and falls, such infections do not cause heart slowing.

243 B

The survival data (inclusion in trial to death) is best described by the medial survival time of the intervention group. The questions related to costs (D & E) are not answerable from a statistical analysis.

244 D

Coin lesion: a single circular opacity seen on CXR – single pulmonary nodule. If the nodule is greater than 15 mm there is a 50% chance of it being a bronchial carcinoma – particularly in an elderly person. Deposits from a distant primary may appear similar. The Honda sign is found at sacral isotopic bone scanning and represents a sacral insufficiency fracture. There is an increase in uptake of tracer in vertical fractures through both sacral alae and a horizontal fracture across the body of the sacrum (normal stress sites in an osteoporotic bone – the sacrum is a common site).

The widow area is slang for the left anterior descending coronary artery. This vessel is frequently involved with athermanous plaques. Occlusion at this site may be fatal. Both cobblestone mucosal appearances and the string sign (of Kantor) are barium follow-through images of the distal ileum involved by stricturing and ulcerating Crohn's disease.

245 B

The only sensible approach in an attempt to clarify Charlie Dreadnought's circumstances is to recommend that he set aside the psychological benefit of his polypharmacy and stop taking numbers of unnecessary tablets (and 'save £££s'). The manufacturer's profits will suffer but his health and finances should improve.

246 B

Rehabilitation goals are an essential part of clinical geriatric medicine and are developed specifically for an individual patient. The use of goals improves overall outcomes. In the management jargon goals need to be SMART – specific, measurable, achievable, realistic and timely. An occupational therapist's contribution to the setting and achievement of the patient's goals is substantial. The other suggestions are spurious.

247 B

The CURB-65 score counts 1 point for each of the following:

> Confusion
> Urea > 7.0
> Respiratory rate > 30
> Blood pressure < 90 systolic or < 60 diastolic
> Age > 65 years

In the vignette the mental state was not given (scores 0) but Jean Collie was over 65, had a tachypnoea over 30, was hypotensive and had a plasma urea concentration > 7.0 leading her to score 4. The CURB-65 score gives an approximate mortality risk:

score	mortality risk %
0–1	< 5
2–3	≤ 10
4–5	15–30

Older patients tend to have baseline urea figures > 7, which automatically scores 2 – this has to be assessed in the overall clinical context.

248 C

An infarct scar may allow the development of a re-entrant ventricular tachy-cardia around the scar. Very low plasma K$^+$ concentrations (≤ 2.0 mmol/L) are more likely to permit a polymorphic VT or ventricular fibrillation. Ventricular rate and resulting BP do not give diagnostic help.

249 A

While any drug may be associated with disturbed transaminases and jaundice, of the choices offered, amiodarone has the most prominent reputation for liver damage. For atorvastatin, volume 63 (March 2012, page 169) of the BNF states that cholestatic jaundice rarely occurs with this chemical.

250 A

Of the 5 choices, constipation is the nearest to a diagnosis, although the 'diag-nosis' begs the question as to an explanation. B to D are functional states, all of which need an explanation for their occurrence.

251 D

There is nothing in the history to prevent one from believing that this man could not have made an autonomous decision after weighing the pros and cons of his arrangements. A decision made by a person with capacity, but which appears unwise, has to be respected.

252 A

The laboratory reported a pure growth of *S pneumoniae* from sputum and blood: both were fully sensitive to penicillin. Mr Smith's treatment was altered to benzylpenicillin as a better drug than the usual CAP antibiotics. Note that 'rusty sputum' is the classical description of sputum related to a pneumococcal lobar pneumonia.

253 B

The dose of digoxin was much too high for an elderly patient. The 8-hour serum digoxin concentration was over twice the therapeutic reference range. A week later, taking only warfarin, Mr Edge felt better: some appetite had returned, his weight had increased by 2.5 kg (no furosemide) and BP had risen to 105/74. By then serum digoxin had fallen and was in the therapeutic reference range. Four weeks after the first visit the patient was established on: digoxin 62.5, furosemide 20, a statin and warfarin.

The dose of digoxin should be judged in the light of the eGFR because dig-oxin is excreted mainly in urine. Cliff Edge's clearance was 32 ml/min/1.73 m^2. A dose of 250 mcg daily is almost invariably too high in an elderly person but is not infrequently found.

254 C

An HbA_{1c} of 9.5% (80) is only compatible with uncontrolled diabetes for 3 or more weeks prior to sampling. The result of an OGGT would provide no additional information. For older people in whom fasting plasma glucose lies between ≥ 6.1 and ≤ 6.9 (intermediate fasting glucose) an OGGT might clarify their glucose tolerance status. Those patients in E – impaired glucose tolerance – have an increased risk of progressing to diabetes and have an increased chance of vascular disease.

255 E

The presence of urinary red blood cells or red blood cell casts suggest renal parenchymal damage. A plasma osmolality in the reference range has no discriminatory value. In the presence of dehydration a healthy kidney will respond by restricting Na^+ excretion – a physiological response with low urinary Na^+ concentrations of < 20 mmol/L. Conversely, a damaged kidney (ARF/AKI) loses the ability to adequately conserve Na^+, which is shown by urinary Na^+ concentrations in excess of 50 mmol/L. Exceptions occur.

256 A

Rinne's test (comparison of the relative effectiveness of sound transmission through the middle ear by air conduction) is positive in health. Choices B to E are an inversion of the correct answers. Thus Rinne's tests for middle ear and not cochlea function. Weber's test – in conductive deafness sound is heard in the better ear and helps identify the better functioning cochlea.

257 D

The data are derived from an elderly woman with a BMI of 35 who clearly paid no attention to her T2DM. The raised ALT indicates liver involvement in the metabolic dysfunction and reflects fatty infiltration.

258 D

There was an interval of about 50 years after Mr Quercus finished boxing before Mrs Quercus noted her husband's brain dysfunction. This long period excluded any boxing-related brain consequence. Bruce Quercus had a cardiovascular past history. The same vascular dysfunction affected his brain. The physical signs were predominantly below the waist. Above the waist there were no true PD signs – vascular Parkinson's is sometimes called lower body Parkinsonism.

A healthy person completes the 'Get Up and Go' test in 10 or fewer seconds (see Answer 98).

259 C

It has recently been shown that antidepressant drugs appear to be non-beneficial as a first-line choice for patients similar to the one outlined in the vignette.

see Rodda J, Walker Z, Carter J Depression in older adults. *BMJ*. 2011; **343**: 691–4.

260 E

There are fewer receptor sites in elderly people. This fact explains the smaller doses needed with increasing age. The age-related reduced rate of warfarin metabolism contributes to the need for smaller doses. Warfarin does not undergo first pass metabolism and is metabolised to inactive compounds which are excreted via the gut. GFR does not influence dosage because neither warfarin (99% albumin bound and therefore not passing into the glomerular infiltrate) nor its breakdown products are renally cleared to any significant effect.

261 D

At the age of 88 years, an ischaemic cardiomyopathy is by far the most likely diagnosis. The investigational data are those of non-specific heart failure. A and E are inherited conditions most unlikely to be present in the eighth decade. Cardiac amyloid (AL variety) is a rare condition usually of the elderly. Chagas' disease – South American trypanosomiasis – is confined to that continent and transmitted by the 'kissing bug'.

262 A

The failure of omeprazole to soothe George Grumble's symptoms is not a red flag feature – it only indicates that the 'indigestion' was not acid suppression sensitive – assuming the tablets were taken.

263 B

Change in financial state is perhaps the least daunting of items but reduction in income with reduction in living standards would not be cheering. The other possibilities are all risk factors for inducing a potentially prolonged grieving process.

264 D

A weighted T1 MRI scan with image reconstruction in the coronal plane gives a good demonstration of the medial temporal lobe structures. When this area of the brain is scanned in health the area is 'full of brain'. In early mental decline there is loss of cortical volume. The maintenance of a MMSE score, but with impairment of higher cortical function, points to a fronto-temporal dementia.

T2-weighted and fluid-attenuated inversion recovery (FLAIR) MRI sequences are very sensitive in demonstrating cerebral white matter ischaemic damage. T1-weighted volumetric sequences demonstrate the presence or absence of volume loss/atrophy.

see Scholt JM *et al*. Suspected early dementia. *BMJ*. 2011; **343**: 634–7.

265 C

Non-threatening silent hallucinations in a person with well-preserved memory and a CT showing global loss are all features of LBD.

AD people have a preserved social façade; those with FTD show disinhibited behaviour, those with SD have day-to-day memory loss of the meaning and understanding of words. Patients with VD have no suggestive patterns of higher cortical dysfunction.

Currently there are perhaps 1 million dementia patients in Great Britain with a conservative overall care cost of > £20 billion. Projections suggest 40% more dements by the mid-2020s and a 150% increase by mid-century.

see Petersen RC. Mild cognitive impairment. *New Engl J Med.* 2011; **364**: 2227–34.
Okie S. Confronting Alzheimer's disease. *New Engl J Med.* 2011; **365**: 1069–72.

266 D

It is most improbable that a dying person requires haematinics despite many of them having some degree of anaemia. If anaemia is symptomatic, a bag of blood gives quick but short-term help. But because a person is anaemic, it does not necessarily follow that treatment is needed. Tissue oxygen requirements of a sedentary person are not great. In the context of Question 266, any desaturation found would be almost certainly a consequence of the lung damage and not from an incidental anaemia.

267 D

Palindromic rheumatism is the only condition that fits Bandleader Mos' symptoms – repeated unpleasant inflammatory attacks of one or two joints. Wrists and small joints of the hands are chiefly involved. The attacks last for only a few hours and up to 48. They tend to occur weekly or up to a single attack every two months. Between attacks the joints are normal. A persistent arthropathy develops in a minority of these people.

268 E

Apart from the therapeutic INR, Mye Badluck fulfilled the criteria for thrombolysis but the addition of rt-PA would have produced an unacceptable, perhaps fatal, degree of anticoagulation. Standard stroke management was appropriate. Most physicians would continue with warfarin. An INR ≥ 1.7 is an exclusion criterion for the use of rt-PA in patients with acute ischaemic stroke.

see Wechsler LR. Intravenous thrombolytic therapy for acute ischaemic stroke. *New Engl J Med.* 2011; **364**: 2138–46.

269 C

The elderly Bea Quick fatally misunderstood Dr Pooter's hurried telephonic advice and she confused the warfarin dose in mg with the number of tablets she needed to take. The pre-mortal INR exceeded 20. The coroner recorded a death by misadventure. The GMC took an unpleasing interest and Dr Pooter was suspended for 3 months and ordered to undergo retraining in drug management.

270 B

The unenhanced brain CT scan showed a compressed distorted brain, age related changes plus hyperdense blood in the subdural space. Hardy Mater had torn a vein or veins that bridge the subdural space. The INR was 2.5, allowing sufficient bleeding to fatally compress the brain.

A torn meningeal artery might well produce a very similar clinical picture – an extradural bleed.

271 A

Some patients with painful terminal disease may need repeated assurance that their latter days will be comfortable and without pain. While patients may ask hospice staff about their religious beliefs, such views should only be expressed when requested – a palliative care facility is not a conversion hunting ground. Different people and their close relatives will have different and perhaps fluctuating views as to where they wish to die.

Spirituality is broadly defined as involving those matters which give a person meaning in life and need not involve any specific religious tenet.

272 B

The presence of leucocyte esterase is a marker for pyuria which is found in 20–30% of 80-year-old healthy women – asymptomatic bacteruria. Such a finding presages a symptomatic urinary tract infection but treatment of the asymptomatic woman does not result in persistently sterile urine. As treatment with synthetic penicillin may result in mucosal candidiasis, diarrhoea and lead to antimicrobial resistance, it should be kept for the symptomatic patient.

The finding of a bacilluria in older men has a similar significance.

The correct clinical decision on the vignette case was not to prescribe antibiotics.

see Hooton TM. Uncomplicated urinary tract infection. *New Engl J Med.* 2012; **366**: 1028–37.

273 C

Sid Weal was obliged to notify DVLA because of his post-stroke central processing deficit. There is a medical section of DVLA the staff of which make individual decisions based on medical reports. Mr Weal's slowness of mind suggested a lack of fitness to drive.

see www.dvla.gov.uk;medicalrules

274 D

It was essential that Mrs Jones was taken to a safe place and treated by people who were trained in the correct procedures. Social Service staff were able to activate a sexual molestation team the members of which included a trained sexual assault examiner and a rape crisis counsellor who explained choices available and discussed matters with family and friends. If sexual assault was established and charges pressed, the police would attempt to capture the perpetrator.

There are time limits for evidence collection; Mrs Jones should not have been offered a shower until forensic material had been collected. The posterior structures of the female external genitalia are most frequently damaged in cases of penetrative rape. The use of post-exposure HIV prophylaxis is controversial when the criminal is unknown.

see Linden JA. Care of the adult patient after sexual assault. *New Engl J Med.* 2011; **365**: 834–41.

275 B

Currently the correct recommendation is to remeasure the BP in 3–4 weeks but some advocate obtaining a 24-hour BP record. This is ideal but expensive in time and money. Concerning options D and E – the prescription of BP-lowering drugs without bothering to determine whether the patient is hypertensive would be poor medical practice even though the choice of drugs is NICE (2011) compliant.

see Richie LD, Campbell NC, Murchie P. New NICE guidelines for hypertension. *BMJ.* 2011; **343**: 491–2.

276 E

Incontinence is a frequent feature of fits, but not of other acute loss of consciousness events.

see Leung ES. Funny turns. *BMJ.* 2011; **343**: 1222–3.

277 C

A Pancoast's tumour grows and involves the left recurrent laryngeal nerve (hoarse voice, dysphonia, bovine cough), compression of the sympathetic ganglion causing an ipsilateral Horner's syndrome (ptosis, meiosis (sunken eye) and ipsilateral anhydrosis). Exophthalmos is a protrusion of an eye as in Graves's disease and has no association with a Pancoast's tumour.

278 E

Restless legs are an infrequent but well-recognised side-effect of quetiapine treatment. A dry mouth is a consequence of taking an atypical antipsychotic drug – an antimuscarinic effect.

279 C

Without brain imaging, antiplatelet or anticoagulant drugs should not be used. The patient was transferred to a neighbouring hospital.

280 A

Presbyopia (long-sightedness) is part of normal ageing beginning during middle age. 20/20 and 6/6 vision mean the same. The numerator (the top number) is a standard distance of 6 m (more often used in Britain) or 20 ft (more often used in USA). During vision testing, statement C is measured, leading to a numerical expression of visual acuity.

281 C

The laboratory data indicate Paget's disease (osteitis deformans) – this is often asymptomatic but may cause pressure-related symptoms. Fractures and secondary cancer deposits would be painful. Osteosarcoma is predominantly a tumour of childhood or adolescence – when it occurs in later life it is usually a complication of Paget's. Osteomalacia is associated with high alkaline phosphatase, low or low normal serum Ca^{2+}, low vitamin D and raised PTH.

282 A

It was essential to know whether the woman had advanced renal parenchymal damage (kidneys circa 8.0 cm bipolar length, or less) or obstruction to the flow of urine (renal stones, bladder cancers catching ureters at their insertion). An ultrasound study showed two 10.5 cm kidneys (normal lengths). With intravenous saline the serum creatine fell to the reference range and the woman with a diagnosis of dehydration (pre-renal failure) returned to her nursing home.

283 C

An outgoing attitude and activity help the bereaved person to reorganise and adjust their lives to their loss. Of bereaved persons, elderly widowers have the highest rate of successful suicide.

284 C

The combination of median temporal lobe and hippocampal atrophy is very suggestive of Alzheimer's disease. The shrinking brain (cortical atrophy) allows the development of ventricular dilation and widened (enlarged) sulci but such findings are non-specific.

285 C

Primary hyperparathyroidism is often a chronic benign condition in elderly women, the majority of whom do not require surgery. At 86, Mrs Strongbone is unlikely to be disadvantaged by a mildly raised serum calcium. Annual bone densitometry and serum calcium assay is usually recommended for robust octogenarians. See also Answer 40.

see Pallan S. Diagnosis and management of primary hyperthyroidism. *BMJ*. 2012; **344**: 55–60.

286 D

Onycholysis may be associated with psoriasis, fungal infection, over-or under-active thyroid states, the use of psoralens and local trauma. No explanation is found in most patients.

287 B

While the patient was probably mentally disabled it would have been incorrect to assume that there was necessarily loss of capacity. Thus formal assessment of capacity was the first and correct step.

288 E

A speech and language therapist (SALT) was able to define the extent of the difficulty and advise on the most suitable, at least short-term, feeding strategy. D and B may be appropriate subsequently.

289 B

The noise of tinnitus is generated from the auditory pathways – cochlea, VIII cranial, brain stem or auditory cortex – after damage or injury. An explanation for the condition is often not found. Tinnitus often accompanies deafness and is one of a triad of symptoms in Ménière's disease – tinnitus, vertigo and deafness. High-dose intravenous furosemide may induce reversible tinnitus.

290 B

The clue to the diagnosis was the development of a rash and chest symptoms with a diffuse hemisphere process following a number of fractures. A, C and E would have been associated with abnormalities of the CSF – at least elevation of protein content.

In some people who fracture a number of bones, fat globules escape into the systemic circulation. The usual sites of embolisation are the skin of the anterior upper torso, lungs and brain.

291 E

The LVEF is calculated from the difference in left ventricular volume between maximum filling and the end of systole. There is always a residual ventricular volume; hence maximum function cannot be 100%. The measurements from which the LVEF is calculated depend upon the quality of the left ventricular ultrasound images, which at times are less than ideal. LVEF results are:

>55%	normal
46–55	mild impairment
35–45	moderate impairment
< 34	severe impairment
< 25	approaching terminal left ventricular failure

292 B

Richard Bright had developed an acute thrombosis of his superior sagittal sinus as shown by the hyperdense image obtained from its lumen (the hyperdense cord sign).

A hyperdense image indicates fresh clot, an old clot appears hypodense compared with the surrounding brain.

Precipitating factors of venous thrombosis include dehydration, the OCP, prednisolone and hypercoagulable states which include nephrotic syndrome.

293 B

The Ishihara colour plate is a test of colour vision and not visual acuity assessment. If the top line of a Snellen chart cannot be read at 1 m, the subject should be asked to count fingers. If that fails, can hand movements be detected? If that too fails, the last test is whether light can be perceived.

294 A

While B to E are correct, they stem from an appreciation of GFR – usually expressed as eGFR.

295 D

Because the 'D' patient was putting on a brave face in adversity, that was no reason to reduce the frequency of routine observations which may have been to his advantage.

296 E

Norovirus has become an important public health matter, usually occurring in closed communities such as hospitals, homes for the elderly, schools and cruise ships. Incubation is 15–50 hours. The onset is typically with acute gut upset and with a three-day resolution. The attack rate is very high with a low infective dose.

297 D

The different appearances are reflections upon the following:
  A T2-weighted FLAIR sequences are very sensitive for cerebrovascular disease
  B these changes reflect a limbic encephalitis
  C well suggestive of fronto-temporal lobe degeneration
  D these findings in a person with isolated memory impairment has a substantial predictive value for subsequent development of AD
  E such images suggest mixed vascular cognitive impairment and AD

see Grodstein F. How early can cognitive decline be detected? *BMJ*. 2012; **344**: 10.

298 A

Best Banting could have been sodium depleted due to the thiazide indapamide. Stopping this drug was the first step in managing the 40/8 mm Hg postural drop.

299 D

Given the seniority of the prescriber one can assume that the diagnosis was correct and suitable drugs in adequate doses were being prescribed. Inadequate compliance is a possibility: if the patient is not forthcoming or cannot remember tablet taking, having plasma drug concentrations measured should clarify matters. A dosette box and some supervision of medicine taking can be valuable.

300 A

NICE guidelines (2010) concluded that there was no evidence to favour A over B or vice versa. More recent studies suggest that daily tiotropium has an edge in symptom control (The POET-COPD trial 2011). Trial results of combining tiotropium and salmeterol (choice E) have not been reported.

see Wedzicha JA. Choice of bronchodilator treatment for patients with COPD. *New Engl J Med.* 2011; **364**: 1167–8.

Siafakas NM. Preventing exacerbations of COPD. *New Engl J Med.* 2011; **365**: 758–4.

301 A

Patients in whom AF is, has been, or may be present, have an equal risk of developing an embolic stroke. The CURB-65 score is a risk assessment tool for patients with pneumonia; not heart conditions. The use of warfarin carries a slightly greater risk than that for aspirin use, but is superior to aspirin in stroke prevention (see Answer 329). An INR of 3–4 is not superior in terms of prevention of atrial emboli to an INR of 2–3.

For octogenarians and their seniors, stroke prevalence is 10%.

Paroxysmal AF = episodes that terminate spontaneously within one week; persistent AF = failure to terminate spontaneously within one week; permanent AF = the arrythmia lasting more than one year.

see Khoo CW, Lip GYH. Atrial fibrillation. *Medicine.* 2010; **38**: 507–14.

302 E

Assuming the patient was not allergic to penicillins, intravenous (IV) flucloxacillin was the drug of first choice. Some also use IV benzyl penicillin for the duration of the flucloxacillin therapy. Oral flucloxacillin with or without phenoxymethyl penicillin are poor second choices for hospitalised patients. For those allergic to, or thought to be allergic to, penicillins either IV clindamycin or clarithromycin are used, the choice being decided by local antibiotic policy.

The very low IgG concentration was suggestive of an immune paresis favouring aggressive infections.

303 B

Uncle Tom had spent many hours in the open, so it was not surprising that he developed a basal cell carcinoma (rodent ulcer). These tumours grow slowly and have well-demarcated edges which often take on a 'rolled' appearance. They do not metastasise.

Squamous cell carcinomas also occur on sun-exposed areas, ulcerate and have irregular edges. They may metastasise. Malignant melomata grow rapidly as a pigmented nodule; they may bleed and ulcerate. They metastasise. The nodular variety is the most aggressive. The superficial spreading malignant melanoma is flat and irregularly pigmented with irregular edges. It is the most common. The amelanotic variety is the least common, but very dangerous.

304 A

The Bristol classification of stools ranges from 1 (hard to pass pellets) to type 7 – entirely liquid. Active CD infection and the passage of a Bristol type 1 to 2 is oxymoronic. In health the daily stool volume is around 200 ml. CD toxin is excreted for four or more weeks after the infection has settled clinically.

see Shannon-Lowe J, Matheson NJ, Cooke FJ, Aliyu SH. Prevention and medical management of *Clostridium difficile* infection. *BMJ*. 2010; **340**: 641–6.

305 E

A to D are well-recognised features of a diabetic autonomic neuropathy; postural hypotension being the most frequent. Other neuropathic manifestations are impotence, absent sweating, urinary retention, altered papillary reflexes and a fixed heart rate. Diabetic foot ulcers are a feature of a peripheral neuropathy which is present in 80% of such cases – the lowered awareness of pain/trauma/stones in shoes allowing skin damage. Peripheral vascular disease and microvascular circulatory disease lead to local ischemia. Anhydrosis on the basis of autonomic neuropathy allows the skin to crack, giving a portal of entry for bacteria. Diabetic ulcers may occur anywhere on the foot, but are common at the tips of claw and hammer toes and metatarsal heads.

306 D

Mrs Thinbones was very vitamin D deficient and was at distinct risk of a fracture of her osteoporotic bones. Her impaired mobility was explained by weak quadriceps – a feature of vitamin D deficiency. Prolonged treatment with calcium, vitamin D and a bisphosphonate improved gait speed and reduced the risk of falls and fractures.

see Rosen CJ. Vitamin D insufficiency. *New Engl J Med*. 2011; **364**: 248–54.

307 E

The converse is true for points A, B and C. The AA is claimable from a client's 65th birthday onwards. Retrospective claims are not considered. The AA, like many other benefits available for older people, is not claimed as often as it could because a potential claimant is often unaware of its existence, is confused by the application process or prefers not to receive 'charity money'.

308 E

A fasting plasma glucose of ≥ 7.0 or a random non-fasting figure of ≥ 11.1 establishes the diagnosis. Mrs Sugar was obviously diabetic and therefore the figures of 3.0, 5.5 and 6.9 were spurious. The obesity and duration of symptoms were easily compatible with a plasma glucose figure of 17.2.

309 E

This man had a typical history of benign paroxysmal positional vertigo (BPPV). The physical signs were elicited by the Hallpike test (a test of labyrinthine function). BPPV is the most common cause of intermittent vertigo. It may follow infection or head trauma. It is caused by crystals of calcium carbonate settling within the endolymphatic fluid of the semi-circular canals. The condition is self-limiting but may be recurrent. Ménière's disease causes non-positional vertigo.

310 A

A hypoxic (syncope-affected brain) may well produce discharges that cause twitches or fits. To a non-experienced viewer the sight of a syncope-related convulsion would not differentiate it from a true seizure. B to E are generally more diagnostically useful. Those with cardiac syncope have an annual attrition rate (mortality) of about 10%. Cardiovascular syncope is far more common than epilepsy and they may be very difficult to distinguish from each other.

see Leung ES. Funny turns. *BMJ*. 2011; **343**: 1222–3.

311 C

When the hand is at the level of the greater trochanter, the elbow is at 15–20° of flexion. This allows the most efficient muscular function of the elbow. Mobility is increased by transmitting some of the body's weight through the arm, thereby diminishing the static forces on the affected hip or knee.

The top of the handle to the tip of the ferrule should equal the distance from the proximal wrist crease to ground when the subject is standing in his shoes and the elbow flexed to about 20°. This allows the stick to be placed ahead when walking.

A horizontal handle of a walking stick is preferred because with a curved handle pressure is concentrated on a small area on the base of the palm.

see Mulley GP. *Everyday Aids and Appliances.* London: BMJ; 1989.

Mulley GP. *More Everyday Aids and Appliances.* London: BMJ; 1991.

312 C

Mrs Pill was critically ill, as shown by liver and kidney dysfunction, deranged coagulation and acidosis with much raised lactate. Over the period Christmas to January 1st an excessive amount of paracetamol had unknowingly been consumed. For 36 hours before death she was too ill to take any medication, explaining the low serum paracetamol concentration. Liver injury was increased because phenytoin is an enzyme-inducing drug. Mrs Pill's fatal error was in not appreciating that the proprietary medicine contained paracetamol, thus almost doubling the normal daily dose. The coroner recorded an accidental death.

313 D

Examples of the drugs A to E are haloperidol, clozapine, chlorpromazine, rasagiline and domperidone, respectively.

There is trial work clearly showing that MAO-B drugs (rasagiline and selegiline) delay the progression of parkinsonism. They function by extending the activity of such dopamine that is still secreted and may be used to delay the start of dopa therapy.

314 D

A dose of 120 to 180 mg will be needed. Diuretics have to reach renal tubular lumens to block Na^+ excretion and induce a diuresis. Most diuretics are organic acids. In renal failure there is renal retention of endogenous organic acids. The exogenous organic acid furosemide has to compete with the endogenous acids to enter tubular fluid for it to function as a diuretic. Thus the need for higher doses (and the failure of smaller doses) when the GFR is reduced.

315 A

Rosiglitazone and pioglitazone are contraindicated in patients with heart failure or history thereof. There is only one available biguanide – metformin – which Mr Big cannot tolerate because of nausea and diarrhoea. The sulphonylureas include gliclazide. It would have been unlikely to gain glycaemic control by swapping to a second drug of the same class. Sitagliptin increases insulin secretion and decreases glucagon secretion. It is licensed to be used with either a biguanide or sulphonylurea in patients of European origin with T2DM and a BMI > 35 (NICE).

see Wilding JPH, Hardy K. Glucagon-like peptide-1 analogues for T2DM. *BMJ.* 2011; **342**: 433–6.

316 E

Basal creps are present in many elderly people and their presence is not necessarily obviously pathological. In a person with a BMI of 32 the neck will be so fat that the jugular veins would not be visible.

Blood urea is difficult to interpret because it is affected by fever, food, renal function and starvation. A change in serum creatinine concentration may reflect a change in renal venous back pressure but would be difficult to adequately interpret. An echocardiogram is often of help but is not sensitive to changes of early left ventricular failure and is difficult to arrange quickly in an acute or outpatient setting. Pro-BNP is the measurement of choice because it provides the highest sensitivity and specificity for diagnosing or excluding left heart failure. If the BNP concentration is < 400 ng/L heart failure is unlikely; if > 1000, LVF is very probable. Serial BNP figures may be used to help assess treatment.

317 D

A to C are desirable to give the best support. Neuroleptics – antipsychotic drugs – phenothiazines (prochlorperazine) and butyrophenones (haloperidol) are best avoided in the elderly. Antipsychotics are associated with an increased risk of mortality, stroke, TIA, hypotension and impairment of body temperature regulation in extremes of ambient temperature. Additionally, parkinsonian symptoms, tardive dyskinesia (Answer 210) and the neuroleptic malignant syndrome (Answer 184) are possible sequelae.

318 A

Matters are entirely satisfactory; no immediate additional steps were needed. While diagnostically correct and desirable, it is often very difficult to successfully achieve a temporal artery biopsy.

319 A

The 2011 NICE guidelines classify inadequately controlled blood pressure as 'resistant hypertension' if the subject is taking an ACEI, CCB and thiazide. The fourth-step suggestions are to add spironolactone, an α-blocker, a β-blocker or 'higher doses of thiazide-like diuretic'. There is no discussion as to how to convince an asymptomatic person to take, long-term, four separate chemicals to achieve pressure control. The 'poly pill' may have a place in this circumstance.

see Krause T. Management of hypertension. Summary of NICE guidelines. *BMJ*. 2011; **343**: 474–6.

320 E

After a month the patient was grateful to be placed in a respite facility while B was being performed.

321 B

There are two features in the vignette strongly supporting the diagnosis: the rapid weight increase with resulting median nerve compression, and the easing overnight manoeuvres.

Carpal tunnel syndrome is a complication of sub-thyroid states (A).

322 C

A Mobitz type II trace indicates a significant myocardial abnormality which has a high chance of progression to complete heart block. A prophylactic pacemaker implant was essential.

A, B, D and E are all normal findings and were discarded in making the diagnosis.

323 B

While all of A to E are possible consequences of giving a β-blocker to a man with COAD, it has recently been appreciated that the probability of benefit easily outweighs the risk of harm. Bisoprolol is a logical drug to use in Brian Fagg's management because of his cardiovascular disease. Beta-blocking drugs reduce overall deaths from cardiovascular disease and, surprisingly, respiratory morbidity may also be reduced.

324 C

The risk is 'medium' because the ABCD2 system reaches a score of 4. Such scoring does not have 'minor' or 'critical' subdivisions. The risk is calculated from:

	features		points
A	age	> 60	1
B	BP	≥ 140/90	1
C	clinical features	unilateral weakness	2
		only speech disturbed	1
D	duration of dysfunction	≥ 60 minutes	2
		10–59 minutes	1
2	diabetes		1

From the vignette data, the score is 4. This puts the patient in the low-risk group – 0 to 3 points compared with medium-risk 4 to 5 and high-risk 6 to 7. A score of 4 or more constitutes a medical emergency needing immediate help.

325 B

A clinical diagnosis was not possible but the CRP and white cell count suggested infection. Biochemical results showed a non-obstructive hepato-biliary event (had the alkaline phosphatase been from bone, one would have expected a localising symptom or sign). Ampicillin is now the antibiotic of first choice in biliary sepsis, having replaced cephalosporins because of the risk of inducing *C difficile* overgrowth.

326 B
While neonatal survival may be increasing, these children have no bearing on the longevity of those in their eighth decades and more. Factors A and C to E are contributing to the increasingly elderly population of Great Britain. Currently, almost 16% of the UK population are aged 65+ years and there are more people > 60-years-old than < 16 years. The 2012 UK population is 62.5 million.

327 C
The forward bowing of the tibiae, the 'cotton wool' skull changes and the pseudofractures in the tibiae with the isolated elevation of alkaline phosphatase are all characteristic of an advanced case of Paget's disease of bone. The condition is a fairly common disorder of bone architecture which occurs with increasing frequency after middle age. At first there is bone reabsorption, followed by uncoordinated repair. The reparative process leads to deposition of disorganised bone with abnormal modelling and deformity. The pseudofractures are incomplete fractures found on concave surfaces of bowed bones.

328 C
It is probable that this woman had infected urine. Trimethoprim was the antibiotic of choice. With control of the toxaemia of infection, the heart rate settled spontaneously.

329 E
Suggestions A to D are wrong. The benefit of warfarin anticoagulation is as stated in E. The target INR is 2.5 – persistently less than that provides no protection and > 3 increases the risk of bleeding. Both persistent and paroxysmal AF are strong predictors of first and recurrent brain attack. Warfarin is substantially more efficacious than aspirin and should be used accordingly.

see Garge BF. Cost of dabigatran for atrial fibrillation. *BMJ*. 2011; **343**: 915–16.

330 A
An evening diuresis, completed before retiring and with the avoidance of a bedtime drink would render Mrs Small-Puddle relatively dehydrated and thus reduce her nocturia – this is helpful in some. An evening thiazide dose would be ineffective and at any time is not a suitable drug for a person with nocturia. DDVAP might be of value; it is unlicensed for use in the elderly. The use of TCA needed to be reconsidered because of potential postural hypotension and overnight sedation – a fall-risking combination.

331 B

The patient has crossed physical signs. The lesion cannot therefore be cortical. Crossed signs tend to reflect a brainstem lesion. In Question 331 the left brainstem was implicated – LMN signs (facial droop) from the VII cranial nerve with right UMN signs – corticospinal tract damage causing the right hemiplegia.

332 E

The rhythm trace showed normal atrial and QRS activity, but showed gaps (pauses) when there was no atrial impulse passing to the ventricles. Normal P-wave activity then resumed, leading to normal QRS complexes. This is the sick sinus syndrome, a cause of collapse and a prelude to asystole. A pacemaker had to be inserted urgently.

333 C

Chlortalidone is a thiazide-related compound and has the same side-effects including hyponatraemia, hypokalaemia, hyperglycaemia and hyperuricaemia as all thiazides. The other four drugs may all be implicated in hyponatraemia (as SIADH-inducing agents) but do not additionally affect potassium, glucose and urate metabolism.

334 B

Despite the normal bone structure demonstrated by x-ray, osteomyelitis was not excluded. Arterial supply to the foot seemed satisfactory, as judged by the normal APBI (1.1). MRI is more sensitive than CT in demonstrating infected bone changes – choices D and E were not needed.

335 C

It is impossible to practice geriatric medicine without an appreciation of colonic dysfunction – constipation with or without overflow (often misdiagnosed as diarrhoea) is very frequently found in wards and out-patient clinics. On a back pressure basis, from a constipated colon, anorexia, nausea and vomiting may be mis-diagnosed as bowel obstruction. Pains are frequent in the elderly and opiate analgesia is often required with under-recognised stool stagnation.

Endocrine disease may either present via the large gut or affect the gut in the later stages.

336 A

Systemic infection is not a recognised cause of onycholysis. In this condition the nail separates from its bed distally and spreads proximally before detaching. Dysmorphic regrowth then occurs.

Psoralens are plant products which make the skin temporally sensitive to ultraviolet as part of treatment of psoriasis.

337 D

The vignette contains insufficient information to learn whether stopping the hypotensive drugs proved sufficient and whether the patient had an autonomic neuropathy contributing to the postural drop.

T2DM, unlike T1DM, is not known to have an autoimmune background and there is no recognised link with autoimmune adrenal failure. Hence to ask for adrenal antibodies to be assayed would have been illogical.

see Sathyapalan T, Aye MM, Atkin SL. Postural hypotension. *BMJ*. 2011; **343**: 39–41.

338 E

As the elderly male population increases, so does the incidence and prevalence of malignant prostatic disease. Nevertheless, the overall prognosis is generally good; many men require no treatment – those with this tumour usually die of different causes. Options A to D are correct consequences of the expanding discipline of the health of older people.

339 B

From the history it was likely that Wm Flowerdew had bladder outflow obstruction (BOO). A DRE cannot assess accurately the effect of BPH on the urethra. A bladder scan clarified matters. If a residual had been present an α-adrenoceptor agonist or a 5α-reductase inhibitor would have been helpful for the BOO symptoms.

Apart from inconvenience, nocturia is a risk factor for falls, bone fracture, daytime somnolence and enuresis.

340 D

The clinical picture was that of acute closed-angle glaucoma. This results from obstruction to the outflow of aqueous humor at the iris. Intraocular pressure increases, distorting vision, and is measured by tonometry to confirm the clinical diagnosis.

Conversely, open-angle glaucoma is asymptomatic, often diagnosed at routine eye examination. It is more common than the closed-angle variety.

341 A

The ischaemic chest pain, hypotension and bradycardia imply inadequate peri-infarct arterial perfusion as a consequence of the bradycardia of excessive vagal tone. Thus atropine (an anticholinergic drug) was needed urgently to reduce vagal tone, allowing an increase in ventricular rate, improved left ventricular ejection fraction and improved coronary perfusion of all parts of the myocardium.

342 C

This man fitted the core diagnostic features of fronto-temporal dementia and demonstrates the complexity of the diagnostic process. Pick's disease is a histological subdivision of FTD.

The core criteria of FTD are:

1. insidious onset with slow progression
2. early:
   i. decline in social interpersonal conduct
   ii. impairment of control of personal conduct
   iii. emotional blunting
   iv. loss of insight
3. together with: reduction in personal hygiene/grooming, mental rigidity, distractibility, change in food likes, stereotyped behaviour

343 C

Sucralfate is a complex of aluminium hydroxide and sucrose which, while having minimal antacid properties, has a barrier function that gives gastric mucosal protection.

The other four compounds reduce H^+ secretion. Bacteria are less likely to colonise the stomach when the pH is above normal. Sick patients may aspirate such bacteria. Less gastric colonisation occurs when sucralfate is used.

344 B

Medicine has become increasingly complex such that a practitioner in say, GiM, cannot be expected to have broad-spectrum medical detail at his finger tips. Thus guidelines drawn up by committees of experts – as per NICE or specialist groups such as the British Thoracic Society – are available to supply generalists with accurate contemporary information.Guidelines are broad statements from which specific clinical decisions are made and implemented.

There is some truth in A, C and E.

345 C

Dermal loss only is a Waterlow Class II. The correct treatment involves:

the ulcer being kept clean;
the ulcer being kept moist;
the avoidance of topical antibiotics;
repeated changes of position of an adequately nourished patient.

Answer 49 has a classification of ulcer severity.

see NICE. *The Prevention and Treatment of Pressure Sores.* NICE Clinical Guideline 29. London: NICE; 2005.
see www.nice.org.uk/cg29

346 D

The MMSE score must be between 15 and 20 to justify a trial of treatment. If introduced at a score of 25, there would be no discernable change.

see Schneider LS. Discontinuing donezipil or starting memantine for Alzheimer's disease? *New Engl J Med.* 2012; **366**: 957–9.

347 B

The majority of lesions that disturb production or comprehension of speech and language lie in the dominant hemisphere. The left hemisphere is dominant in about 95% of right-handed people. Thus for Mr Boxgrove the lesion was in the left and probably in the posterior frontal lobe along the insula and Sylvian fissure and not only in Broca's area. Blood supply is from the left middle cerebral artery.

348 C

To dispatch this poor man to anywhere without some weeks of rehabilitation would have been very poor management. Eight weeks of intensive mobility relearning and self-caring skills set up the man for a further 3 years of happy independent living until he died acutely in his daughter's home in Santiago.

349 A

A number of placebo-controlled RCTs have shown that in patients with NYHA III or IV dyspnoea of heart failure origin and who are treated with β-blockers, there is:

> a 35% reduction mortality and
> a reduced need for heart failure related admissions.

The benefits are in addition to those from background ACEI medication. Bisoprolol or nebivolol are generally used. The COPD would be expected to improve and the T1DM be unaffected.

see Waller DG, Waller JR. Beta-blockers for heart failure with reduced ejection fraction. *BMJ.* 2011; **343**: 691–4.

350 D

This elderly man was frail and mentally compromised. Non-invasive management of his iron-deficient anaemia was correct. If there difficulties with tablet consumption, no treatment would have been an acceptable decision – choice C. Before prescribing, one would need to consider the aim of iron therapy – for the benefit of an asymptomatic person or as a consequence of the prescriber's semi-automatic response?

The man was bed-bound; his anaemia was asymptomatic since the limited need for much tissue delivery of oxygen. Ferrous sulphate is perhaps the most widely over-prescribed drug in geriatric practice.

Index

T - #0669 - 101024 - C0 - 246/174/10 - PB - 9781846195761 - Gloss Lamination